ORTHOPAEDIC
POCKET
PROCEDURES

ORTHOPAEDIC POCKET PROCEDURES

FOOT AND ANKLE

ARMEN S. KELIKIAN, MD

Associate Professor of Orthopaedic Surgery
Northwestern University Medical School
Chicago, Illinois

Series Editor

COURTLAND G. LEWIS, MD

Clinical Professor of Orthopaedic Surgery
University of Connecticut School of Medicine
Farmington, Connecticut

Illustrator

TIMOTHY E. HENGST

McGRAW-HILL
MEDICAL PUBLISHING DIVISION

New York   Chicago   San Francisco
Lisbon   London   Madrid   Mexico City   Milan
New Delhi   San Juan   Seoul   Singapore
Sydney   Toronto

ORTHOPAEDIC POCKET PROCEDURES: FOOT AND ANKLE
Copyright © 2004 by **The McGraw-Hill Companies, Inc.** All rights
reserved. Printed in the United States of America. Except as permitted
under the United States Copyright Act of 1976, no part of this publica-
tion may be reproduced or distributed in any form or by any means, or
stored in a data base or retrieval system without the prior written per-
mission of the publisher.

1 2 3 4 5 6 7 8 9 0 DOC/DOC 0 9 8 7 6 5 4 3

ISBN   0-07-136990-2

This book was set in Times Roman by PV&M Publishing Solutions.
The editors were Darlene Cooke and Lisa Silverman.
The production supervisor was Sherri Souffrance.
Project management was provided by Andover Publishing Services.
The index was prepared by Andover Publishing Services.
RR Donnelley was printer and binder.

This book was printed on acid-free paper.

Library of Congress Cataloging-in-Publication Data

Foot and ankle / edited by Armen S. Kelikian.
     p.;cm.—(Orthopaedic pocket procedures)
   Includes bibliographical references and index.
   ISBN 0-07-136990-2
    1. Foot—Surgery—Handbooks, manuals, etc.   2. Ankle—
Surgery—Handbooks, manuals, etc.   I. Kelikian, Armen S.
II. Series.
    [DNLM: 1. Foot—surgery—Handbooks.   2. Ankle—surgery—
Handbooks.   3. Orthopedic Procedures—methods—Handbooks.
WE 39 F6867 2004]
RD563.F635 2004
617.5′85—dc22   2003059291

**CPT codes, descriptions, and material only are Copyright @2001
American Medical Association. All Rights Reserved. No fee sched-
ules, basic units, relative values, or related listings are included in
CPT. The AMA assumes no liability for the data contained herein.
Applicable FARS/DFARS restrictions apply to government use.**

This book is dedicated to my family:
Amara, Armen, Jr., Kosta,
and Toula

CONTENTS

CHAPTER NUMBER/TITLE	CPT CODE	PAGE

CONTENTS

IN ALPHABETICAL ORDER

CHAPTER TITLE	CPT CODE	PAGE

PREFACE

Foot and Ankle is part of a series entitled "Orthopaedic Pocket Procedures." The series covers general topics such as general orthopaedics, pediatrics, and sports medicine, as well as subspecialty topics including hand, and foot and ankle.

This book is intended as a portable point-of-care resource. The procedures are coded according to the American Medical Association's CPT system, which serves as the basis for the reporting of and billing for procedures. The CPT codes are cross-referenced with ICD-9 diagnostic codes, which relate to the condition(s) underlying a given procedure.

The format for each chapter includes anatomy and appropriate surgical approaches as well as relevant information about the specific procedure. Alternative treatment options and postoperative management are also outlined, and a limited bibliography is provided with each procedure.

Foot and Ankle is intended for any health-care provider who is treating problems related to the foot and ankle.

ARMEN S. KELIKIAN, MD
Chicago, Illinois
October 2003

ACKNOWLEDGMENTS

I wish to express my gratitude to my assistant, Barbara Morris; to my editors at McGraw-Hill, Darlene Cook and Lisa Silverman; to our artist, Tim Hengst; and to Niels Buessem for his coordination efforts.

ORTHOPAEDIC POCKET PROCEDURES

BONE GRAFT, MINOR

CPT code   20900 bone graft, any donor area; minor or small (e.g., dowel
                              or button)

ICD-9 code   733.82 fracture non-union
                              bone graft supplementaiton for arthrodesis

INDICATIONS

- non-unions
- arthodesis—stress-relieving bone graft
- comminuted fracture with bone loss

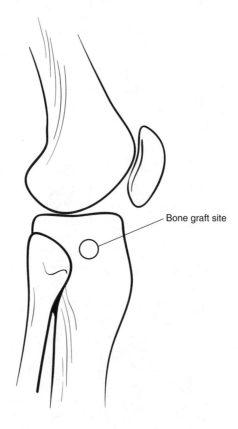

Bone graft site

ALTERNATIVE TREATMENTS

- invasive and noninvasive bone stimulators
- prolonged casting
- Ilizarov small pin ring fixator with bone transport

SURGICAL ANATOMY

Incision

- percutaneous

APPROACHES

- numerous sites include proximal tibia, distal tibia, and distal femur
- posterior and anterior calcaneus

Surgical Techniques

- use hollow reamers, between 6 and 12 mm in diameter (e.g., Spine-Tech and AcroMed)
- metaphyseal bone
- 2-cm incision over Gerdy's tubercle
- penetrate the near cortex with a gentle clockwise motion to a depth of 3 cm
- remove the reamer and use an angled curette to undermine and remove additional cancellous bone
- close the wound

POSTOPERATIVE MANAGEMENT

- non-weight-bearing and immobilization is dictated by the primary procedure, or at least 6 weeks

COMPLICATIONS

- stress fracture

SELECTED REFERENCES

Hansen ST. Functional reconstruction of the foot and ankle. Philadelphia: Lippincott Williams & Wilkins, 2000:490–493.

BONE GRAFT, MAJOR

CPT code   20902 bone graft, major or large

ICD-9 code   733.82 fracture non-union

                    arthrodesis procedures, e.g., subtalar bone block
                    (CPT code 28725)

INDICATIONS

- non-union
- adjunct for arthrodesis procedures
- structural bone graft, e.g., Evans procedure (calcaneal lengthening) (CPT code 28308)

ALTERNATIVE TREATMENTS

- local bone graft (CPT code 20900)
- allograft with or without autogenous growth factor (AGF)
- implantable or external bone stimulator

SURGICAL ANATOMY

Incision

- oblique off the iliac crest, beginning 2 cm posterior to the anterior-superior iliac spine (ASIS) for a length of 4–6 cm

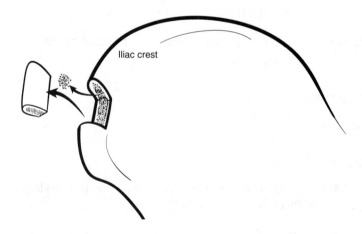

Iliac crest

APPROACHES

Surgical Techniques

- either lateral decubitus (ipsilateral) or with a roll under the buttocks
- the gluteal muscles are elevated from the outer ilium
- a Cobb elevator is used to expose the inner table
- an oscillating microsagittal long-saw blade is used with either large Chandler or Taylor retractors
- the height of the graft determines the second saw cut, usually 1.2 to 2 cm
- the shape and depth of the graft are determined by the angle and length of the saw blade
- a 1-cm curved osteotome is used deep, to complete the resection of the graft
- cancellous bone can be removed from between the tables with angled curettes
- Gelfoam is packed into the void
- the wound is closed in layers

POSTOPERATIVE MANAGEMENT

- compression dressing
- sutures or staples removed at 2 weeks

COMPLICATIONS

- hematoma
- infection
- neuritis: lateral femoral cutaneous nerve
- stress fracture, ASIS

SELECTED REFERENCES

Hansen ST. Functional reconstruction of the foot and ankle. Philadelphia: Lippincott Williams & Wilkins, 2000:485–489.

TENDON GRAFT, FROM A DISTANCE

CPT code   **20924 tendon graft, from a distance**

ICD-9 code   **845 ankle instability**

INDICATIONS

- lack of primary tissue for tendon repair or ligament reconstruction

ALTERNATIVE TREATMENTS

- plantaris versus long-toe extensor

SURGICAL ANATOMY

- fourth long-toe extensor inserts medial to the extensor brevis on the extensor hood; take care to identify and protect branches of the superficial peroneal nerve

Incision

- 2-cm transverse incision over the fourth metatarsal phalangeal joint is made; suture the distal stump of the extensor digitorum longus (EDL) to the extensor digitorum brevis (EDB); the EDL is cut just proximal to this anastomosis
- identify the EDL of the fourth toe just distal to the extensor retinaculum of the ankle; transect the tendon and remove it at this level (alternatively, a tendon stripper may be employed)

APPROACHES

Surgical Techniques

- the plantaris tendon runs underneath the medial border of the gastrocnemius and inserts into the calcaneus at the point of insertion of the Achilles tendon; through a small medial longitudinal incision at the mid-calf, the plantaris tendon is identified and sectioned—it is extricated and sectioned on the medial side of the distal heel cord

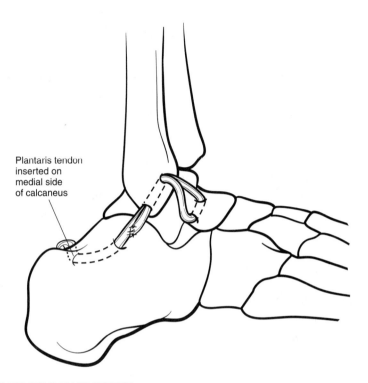

Plantaris tendon
inserted on
medial side
of calcaneus

POSTOPERATIVE MANAGEMENT

- premised on the reconstruction at the recipient site

REHABILITATION

- depends on the primary procedure

COMPLICATIONS

- hammer toe and neuropraxia for EDL free graft

SELECTED REFERENCES

Kelikian AS. Ankle and subtalar instability. In: Kelikian AS, ed. Operative treatment of the foot and ankle. Stamford, CT: Appleton & Lange, 1999: 310–319.

TENDO ACHILLES LENGTHENING

CPT code   27606 tenotomy, percutaneous, Achilles tendon; general anesthesia

ICD-9 code   736.72 equinus deformity of foot, acquired

INDICATIONS

- distal Achilles lengthening is indicated when the ankle cannot be placed in neutral with the knee flexed or extended (Perry test)
- there is no intra-articular or osseous etiology for loss of dorsiflexion

ALTERNATIVE TREATMENTS

- serial stretching casts
- physiotherapy
- dynamic joint jacks
- Botox (neuromuscular causes)

SURGICAL ANATOMY

Incision
- percutaneous via two medial incisions, or two medial incisions and one lateral stab incision

APPROACHES

Surgical Techniques
- the first incision is made 1 cm above the Achilles attachment, just medial and anterior to the heel cord
- the anterolateral fibers are cut while gentle dorsiflexion is applied to the foot
- 4 cm proximal to the first incision, a midline vertical incision is made—the scalpel is directed toward the medial fibers and the foot is dorsiflexed again with the knee extended
- if a third incision is required, it is placed lateral but 2–3 cm above the first incision

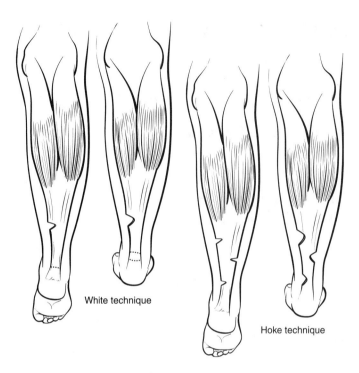

White technique

Hoke technique

POSTOPERATIVE MANAGEMENT

- short-leg cast in 0–5° of dorsiflexion at 2 weeks
- total cast time of 8 weeks
- physiotherapy for strengthening

SELECTED REFERENCES

Hansen ST. Functional reconstruction of the foot and ankle. Philadelphia: Lippincott Williams & Wilkins, 2000:418–420.

NOTES

_____
_____
_____
_____
_____
_____
_____

ARTHROTOMY WITH SYNOVECTOMY, ANKLE

CPT code   **27625 arthrotomy, with synovectomy, ankle**

ICD-9 code   **719.07 unspecified effusion of the ankle joint**

INDICATIONS

- synovitis, not responsive to medical therapy
- infectious arthritis, not responsive to medical treatment

ALTERNATIVE TREATMENTS

- for chronic noninfectious synovitis—nonsteroidal anti-inflammatory drugs (NSAIDs), corticosteroid injection
- septic arthritis—intravenous antibiotics
- arthroscopic synovectomy

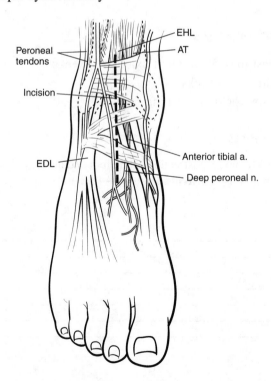

SURGICAL ANATOMY

- majority of synovium can be removed anteriorly, except for the posterior recess

Incision

- anterior longitudinal incision between the interval of the extensor hallucis longus (EHL) and anterior tibial (AT) tendons is developed —care must be taken to protect the superficial peroneal nerve and the neurovascular bundle

APPROACHES

- anterior longitudinal

Surgical Techniques

- the EHL tendon and neurovascular bundle are retracted laterally
- the incision begins 10 cm above the bimalleolar line and extends 5 cm distally—the deep dissection can go lateral to the EHL and the bundle, and medial to the extensor digitorum communis (EDC) alternatively

POSTOPERATIVE MANAGEMENT

- splint in neutral for 2 weeks

REHABILITATION

- range of motion (ROM) at 2 weeks and protected weight-bearing for 2 more weeks

COMPLICATIONS

- neuropraxia of superficial peroneal nerve

SELECTED REFERENCES

Kelikian H, Kelikian A. Disorders of the ankle. Philadelphia: WB Saunders, 1984:170–172.

REPAIR OF ACHILLES TENDON RUPTURE

CPT code   27650 repair, primary, open or percutaneous, ruptured

ICD-9 code   727.67 rupture of Achilles tendon, nontraumatic

INDICATIONS

• active athletic individual, more than 1 cm gap in plantar-flexed position

ALTERNATIVE TREATMENTS

• equinus short-leg cast non-weight-bearing 4 weeks, then 4 weeks weight bearing with a 2-cm heel lift incorporated in walking cast followed by a neutral walking cast

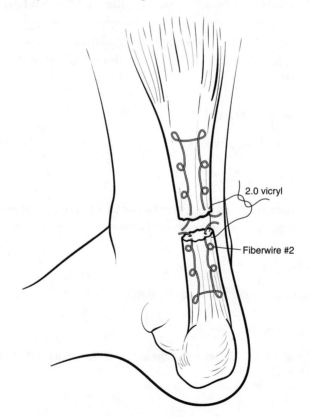

SURGICAL ANATOMY

- the vascularity is poorest in the segment 2–6 cm above the insertion site and contributes to the susceptibility to rupture

Incision
- medial approach just medial to the tendon avoids the sural nerve and allows access to the plantaris tendon if prone; the incision is centered above and below the tear for about 7 cm and should be just anterior to the tendon

APPROACHES

Surgical Techniques
- patient in prone position
- the paratenon is incised along the incision, avoiding dissection between itself and the subcutaneous tissue
- a no. 2 (FiberWire-Arthrex) suture is placed in each limb using a modified Krackow technique; 2 or 4 strands may be used
- after the tendon has been placed in the proper tension the sutures are tied
- a running 3–0 absorbable suture is placed around the repair; the paratenon is closed with a 2–0 absorbable suture; the skin is closed with 3–0 nylon
- if the tear is more proximal, augmentation can be performed with the plantaris or modified Lindholm technique using inverted distal tendon strips

POSTOPERATIVE MANAGEMENT

- equinus splint
- ROM is allowed in plantar flexion mode at 10 days postoperatively
- Bledsoe-type brace with a 1-inch heel lift is applied
- weight bearing is allowed at 5 weeks

REHABILITATION

- strengthening is begun at 6–8 weeks, the brace is maintained until 12 weeks, an elevated heel lift is used for 6 more weeks, and sports are allowed at 9 months

COMPLICATIONS

- re-rupture, 1%
- infection
- skin slough
- sural neuropraxia

SELECTED REFERENCES

Wapner KL. Achilles tendon ruptures and posterior heel pain. In: Kelikian AS, ed. Operative treatment of the foot and ankle. Stamford, CT: Appleton & Lange, 1999:369–387.

NOTES

REPAIR, SECONDARY, ACHILLES TENDON

CPT code   27654 repair, secondary, Achilles tendon, with or without graft

ICD-9 code   727.67 rupture Achilles tendon, nontraumatic

INDICATIONS

- re-rupture or delayed diagnosis

ALTERNATIVE TREATMENTS

- ankle–foot orthosis (AFO)
- peroneus brevis transfer
- allograft

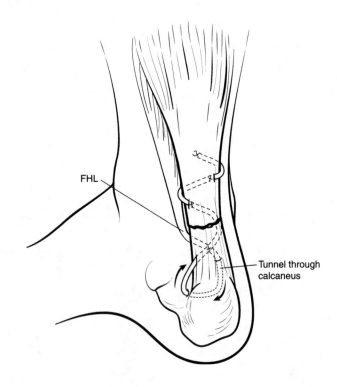

FHL

Tunnel through calcaneus

SURGICAL ANATOMY

- the relationship between the flexor hallucis longus (FHL) and flexor digitorum longus (FDL) (master knot of Henry) for the donor site is critical; the operation can be performed with the patient supine or prone (see figure on page 93)

Incision

- the tendon is approached posteromedial as in a primary repair (CPT code 27650)
- the donor incision is made along the medial border of the foot just above the abductor hallucis from the metatarsal neck to the navicular

APPROACHES

- the abductor hallucis is reflected plantarward with the flexor hallucis brevis; the FHL, which is more superficial, is found and tagged distally; the distal FHL limb is sewn into the FDL; the FHL proximal stump is freed proximally and from all of its attachments with the FDL at the master knot of Henry, and is then delivered throughout the proximal posteromedial incision

Surgical Techniques

- a transverse drill hole (3.5-mm) is made at the Achilles insertion halfway through the calcaneus from medial to lateral; a second drill hole is made vertically to meet the first; the FHL is passed from proximal to the distal with a tendon passer
- after the Achilles has been repaired, the FHL is woven through the Achilles (Pulvertaft weave) with the foot in equinus and tension on the graft; through each weave a suture is placed in the graft and Achilles tendon

POSTOPERATIVE MANAGEMENT

- non-weight-bearing, 15° equinus cast for 4 weeks; the cast is removed and a Bledsoe brace with heel lift is used, similar to rehab protocol for an acute rupture

REHABILITATION

- same as for acute but delayed 4 weeks

COMPLICATIONS

- same as for acute rupture

SELECTED REFERENCES

Kann JA, Meyerson MS. Surgical management of chronic ruptures of the
  Achilles tendon. In: Mandelbaum BR, Myerson MS, eds. Foot and ankle
  clinics: contemporary approaches to the Achilles tendon. Philadelphia:
  WB Saunders, 1997:535–545.

NOTES

_____
_____
_____
_____
_____
_____
_____
_____
_____
_____
_____
_____
_____

REPAIR OF DISLOCATING PERONEAL TENDONS; WITHOUT FIBULAR OSTEOTOMY

CPT code   27675 repair, dislocating peroneal tendons; without fibular osteotomy

ICD-9 code   727.68 other tendons of the foot and ankle

INDICATIONS

- symptomatic instability of the peroneal tendons—chronic

ALTERNATIVE TREATMENTS

- in the acute setting, a non-weight-bearing cast in slight equinus for 4 weeks, followed by a short-leg weight-bearing cast for 4 weeks

SURGICAL ANATOMY

- the superior peroneal retinaculum is the major stabilizing structure for the peronei

Incision
- a longitudinal incision is made over the posterior aspect of the distal fibula

APPROACHES

Surgical Techniques
- if the retinaculum is attenuated, it is incised from the fibula longitudinally to expose the peronei and the sulcus; if the sulcus is shallow it is deepened with a 4-mm burr
- the retinaculum is plicated using biodegradable suture anchors (3.5-mm Panocryl)
- the repair can be augmented with the calcaneofibular (CF) ligament, which is detached from the fibula and brought dorsal to the peronei and then reattached to the fibula

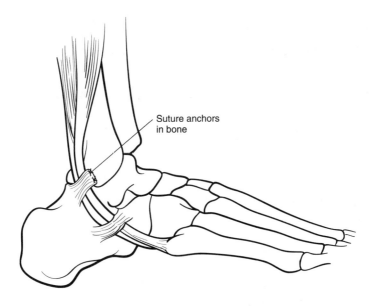

Suture anchors
in bone

POSTOPERATIVE MANAGEMENT

• non-weight-bearing cast 3 weeks, then full-weight-bearing cast
  for 2–3 weeks

REHABILITATION

• avoid forced dorsiflexion and eversion for 8 weeks

COMPLICATIONS

• adhesions and re-subluxation

SELECTED REFERENCES

Leopold SS, Brage ME. Tibialis anterior tendon rupture and peroneal
  subluxation and dislocation. In: Kelikian AS, ed. Operative treatment
  of the foot and ankle. Stamford, CT: Appleton & Lange, 1999:233–254.

REPAIR OF DISLOCATING PERONEAL TENDONS; WITH FIBULAR OSTEOTOMY

CPT code   27676 repair dislocating peroneal tendons; with fibular osteotomy

ICD-9 code   727.68 other tendons of the foot and ankle

INDICATIONS

- symptomatic giving way, snapping, or subjective ankle instability with activity

ALTERNATIVE TREATMENTS

- ankle tapping and bracing are rarely effective
- fibular osteotomy (Kelly bone block)
- calcaneofibular ligament transfer

SURGICAL ANATOMY

- the peroneals evert and plantarflex the foot, and they are maintained over the posterolateral fibula by the peroneal retinaculum in the sulcus; the sulcus is deficient in three-fourths of cases

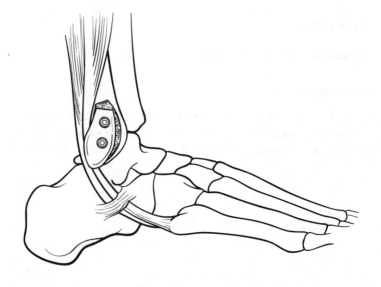

Incision

- longitudinal over the posterior aspect of the distal fibula curving anterior at its tip and avoiding the sural nerve

APPROACHES

Surgical Techniques

- the retinaculum is incised with a periosteal flap off the distal fibula over a 5-cm length; the retinacular flap is based posteriorly
- the tendons and sulcus are inspected for any tears or deficiency
- if the sulcus is shallow, use a 4-mm burr to deepen it
- alternatively, for revision or severe cases, a sagittal osteotomy is made over the lateral third of the distal fibula—a horizontal cut is made 5 cm proximal and the fragment is shifted 5 mm posteriorly
- the retinaculum is repaired by pulling it anteriorly, and attaching it to suture anchors placed at the proximal and distal extent of the reconstructed area along the posterolateral margin of the fibula
- if the retinacular repair is deficient, the calcaneofibular ligament is detached from the fibula and re-routed over the peroneal tendons and then reattached

POSTOPERATIVE MANAGEMENT

- non-weight-bearing coaptation splint for 2 weeks
- short-leg weight-bearing cast for 4 weeks
- short-leg weight-bearing cast for 6 weeks for fibular osteotomy
- ROM and physiotherapy when cast removed
- return to sports at 12 weeks

SELECTED REFERENCES

Leopold SS, Brage ME. Tibialis anterior tendon rupture and peroneal tendon subluxation and dislocation. In: Kelikian AS, ed. Operative treatment of the foot and ankle. Stamford, CT: Appleton & Lange, 1999:233–254.

GASTROCNEMIUS RECESSION, E.G., STRAYER PROCEDURE

CPT code   **27687 gastrocnemius recession (e.g., Strayer procedure)**

ICD-9 code   **727.81 tight heel cords/contracture**

INDICATIONS

- neuromuscular conditions (e.g., cerebral palsy)
- tight heel cord after reconstruction for posterior tibial reconstruction; after realignment the heel cord becomes tighter, since calcaneal valgus and pitch have been improved
- post repair of chronic Achilles rupture
- if the ankle cannot come to neutral with the knee flexed, then a more-distal lengthening is indicated

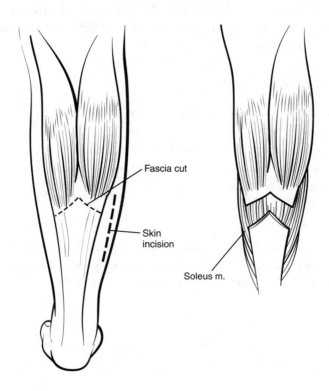

Fascia cut

Skin incision

Soleus m.

ALTERNATIVE TREATMENTS

- night splinting with physiotherapy
- Botox injections for neuromuscular cases
- ankle–foot orthosis (AFO)
- stretching casts
- endoscopic

SURGICAL ANATOMY

Incision
- medial 5 cm between the middle and distal thirds of the leg

APPROACHES

Surgical Techniques
- patient supine or prone
- after subcutaneous dissection, the superficial posterior fascia is incised linearly
- small vaginal speculum or army/navy retractors
- the gastrocnemius aponeurosis is cut like an inverted "V"
- the ankle is dorsiflexed to 7° past neutral
- subcutaneous and skin closure performed

POSTOPERATIVE MANAGEMENT

- short-leg cast, non-weight-bearing for 2 weeks
- short-leg weight-bearing cast for 4 weeks or CAM walker
- physiotherapy and night splinting for 6 more weeks

COMPLICATIONS

- recurrence
- sural neuroma

SELECTED REFERENCES

Hansen ST. Functional reconstruction of the foot and ankle. Philadelphia: Lippincott Williams & Wilkins, 2000.

TRANSFER OR TRANSPLANT OF SINGLE TENDON, SUPERFICIAL

CPT code   **27690** transfer or transplant of single tendon (with muscle redirection/rerouting); superficial (e.g., Girdlestone-Taylor; flexor to extensor transfer)

ICD-9 code   **735.4** claw toes or 2nd IM space syndrome

INDICATIONS

- subluxating or dislocatable second metatarsophalangeal joint
- positive F. Thompson test (Lachman test of the toe)
- not responsive to conservative measures

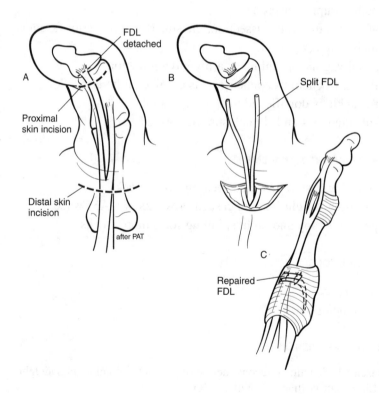

ALTERNATIVE TREATMENTS

- Budin pads
- cross-taping of toe
- extensor brevis transfer for varus crossover of toe

SURGICAL ANATOMY

Incision

- dorsal exposure of the base of the proximal phalanx via a V-shaped incision proximally over the metatarsophalangeal joint, then linear over the toe
- the donor site via two horizontal incisions (interphalangeal and metatarsophalangeal creases) or midline linear incision, plantar

APPROACHES

Surgical Techniques

- after elevating the V flap, the dorsal capsule and collaterals are cut
- if contracted, the extensor tendons are cut as well
- the flexor digitorum longus (FDL) tendon is identified plantar, in between the two limbs of the flexor digitorum superficialis (FDS)
- the bundle is retracted medially and laterally
- the FDL tendon is cut distally
- the two heads are separated at the raphe and then passed subperiosteally and dorsally
- the ankle is placed in 0° of dorsiflexion; the metatarsophalangeal joint in 20° of plantar flexion
- a 1.6-mm K-wire is inserted retrograde to transfix this position
- each arm of the flexor hallucis longus (FHL) tendon is tensioned dorsally and then woven through the extensor mechanism at the base of the proximal phalanx with a 3–0 nonabsorbable suture
- on occasion with a Morton's first ray, a Weil shortening metatarsal osteotomy may be indicated (CPT code 28308)

POSTOPERATIVE MANAGEMENT

- Darco wedge postoperative shoe for 3 weeks
- K-wire removed at 3 weeks, then flat postoperative shoe
- begin passive and active metatarsophalangeal joint exercises when pin removed (10 repetitions, three times per day)

COMPLICATIONS

- stiffness
- recurrence

SELECTED REFERENCES

Watson A, Anderson R, Davis H. Lesser toe deformities. In: Kelikian AS, ed. Operative treatment of the foot and ankle. Stamford, CT: Appleton & Lange, 1999.

NOTES

_____

_____

_____

_____

_____

_____

_____

_____

_____

_____

_____

_____

_____

_____

_____

TRANSFER OR TRANSPLANT OF SINGLE TENDON, DEEP

CPT code   27691 transfer or transplant of single tendon (with muscle redirection or rerouting); deep (e.g., anterior tibial or posterior tibial through interosseous space, flexor digitorum longus, flexor hallucis longus, or peroneal tendon to the midfoot or hindfoot)

ICD-9 code   736.79 foot drop

INDICATIONS

- for peroneal nerve palsy with a deficient anterior tibial tendon; the posterior tibial tendon is transferred through the interosseous membrane and attached to the midfoot centrally
- for a posterior tibial tendon dysfunction, the flexor digitorum longus tendon is transferred to the navicular

ALTERNATIVE TREATMENTS

- ankle–foot orthosis (AFO)
- University of California–Berkeley Laboratory (UCBL) orthosis
- Arizona brace

SURGICAL ANATOMY

- the anterior neurovascular bundle lays in the interval between the tibialis anticus and the extensor hallucis longus; the extensor retinaculum needs to be identified prior to transferring the posterior tibial tendon
- the flexor digitorum longus has its own tunnel just inferior and posterior to the posterior tibial tendon; when addressing posterior tibial dysfunction it can be transferred via a Pulvertaft weave if the posterior tibial tendon is intact or via a drill hole into the navicular

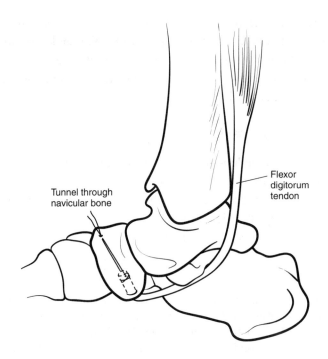

Tunnel through navicular bone

Flexor digitorum tendon

Incision

- posteromedial from the navicular tuberosity to the medial malleolus
- for posterior tibial tendon transfer, an anterior incision is made from a distance of 5–10 cm above the ankle joint just lateral to the crest of the tibia
- the recipient site for the transfer is placed central or lateral with respect to the cuneiforms, depending on the motor balance and strength of the peroneals

APPROACHES

Surgical Techniques

- for posterior tibial tendon transfer, the donor tendon is detached from the navicular and passed around the posterior tibia, then anteriorly through the interosseous membrane; the tendon is then passed over the anterior tibial tendon and beneath the extensor retinaculum
- a suture anchor is placed in the recipient site, and the proper tension is applied with the foot in 5° of dorsiflexion

- for flexor digitorum longus (FDL) transfer, the donor is woven from proximal to distal into the posterior tibial tendon or brought from plantar to dorsal through the navicular drill hole
- Bio-Tenodesis screw (Arthrex) is one means to secure recipient site with proper tension and fixation

POSTOPERATIVE MANAGEMENT

- posterior tibial tendon—6 weeks non-weight-bearing, then 4 weeks full weight-bearing short-leg cast
- FDL transfer—3 weeks non-weight-bearing, then 3 weeks full weight-bearing short-leg cast
- physiotherapy when cast removed

SELECTED REFERENCES

Anderson JG, Hansen ST. Surgical treatment of posterior tibial tendon pathology. In: Kelikian AS, ed. Operative treatment of the foot and ankle. Stamford, CT: Appleton & Lange, 1999:211–234.

Gellmam RE, Anderson RB, Davis WH. Bridle posterior tibial tendon transfer. In: Kitaoka HB, ed. Master techniques in orthopedic surgery: the foot and ankle. Philadelphia: Lippincott Williams & Wilkins, 2002:597–614.

NOTES

_____
_____
_____
_____
_____
_____
_____
_____
_____
_____
_____
_____
_____
_____

REPAIR, PRIMARY, DISRUPTED LIGAMENT, ANKLE; COLLATERAL

CPT code   27695 repair, primary, disrupted ligament, ankle; collateral

ICD-9 code   845.02 sprain calcaneofibular ligament

INDICATIONS

- rare
- results of nonoperative versus operative treatment are equal in the acute setting

ALTERNATIVE TREATMENTS

- functional treatment—proprioception, strengthening, lace-up (Swedo) bracing

SURGICAL ANATOMY

- the anterior talofibular (ATF) and calcaneofibular (CF) ligaments subtend an angle of about 105°; they work in a reciprocal relationship, depending on the ankle position

Incision

- straight, lateral from the tip of the fibula distally for about 5 cm—alternatively, crescent on Langer's lines horizontally submalleolar

APPROACHES

Surgical Techniques

- the peroneal tendons are identified, checked for associated tears, and retracted plantarward
- the CF and ATF ligaments are identified and sutured with 2–0 nonabsorbable suture
- for mid-substance tears: if the ligaments are avulsed from bone, they are reattached with suture anchors; all capsular tears are closed first after joint inspection

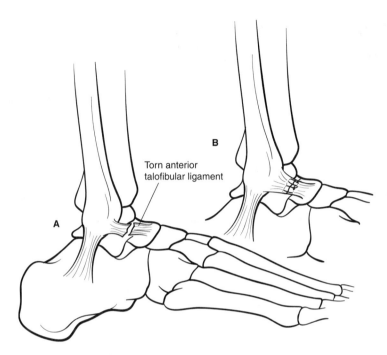

POSTOPERATIVE MANAGEMENT

- non-weight-bearing splint in 5° of eversion and dorsiflexion for 2 weeks, followed by a short-leg weight-bearing cast for 3 weeks

REHABILITATION

- ROM, strengthening, and proprioception exercises when cast removed; lace-up brace is used for protection at this point and when return to athletic activity at 12 weeks

COMPLICATIONS

- neuritis, sural superficial peroneal nerve

SELECTED REFERENCES

Kelikian H, Kelikian A. Disorders of the ankle. Philadelphia: WB Saunders, 1984:472–477.

REPAIR, SECONDARY, DISRUPTED LIGAMENT, ANKLE; COLLATERAL

CPT code   **27698**   repair, secondary, disrupted ligament, ankle, collateral (e.g., Watson-Jones, modified Broström)

ICD-9 code   **845.02** calcaneofibular (ligament) sprain

INDICATIONS

- chronic anterolateral ankle instability, not responsive to conservative measures

ALTERNATIVE TREATMENTS

- bracing, exercises, lateral heel wedges

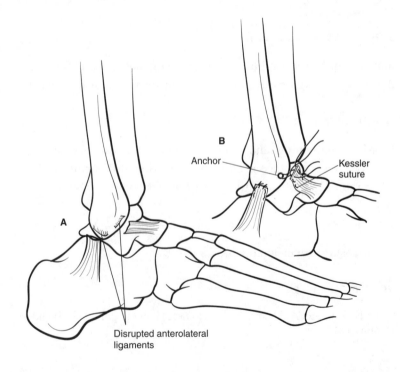

SURGICAL ANATOMY

- the relationship of the anterior talofibular (ATF) and calcaneofibular (CF) ligaments to one another and to the extensor retinaculum

Incision
- straight from the distal fibula for 5 cm distally

APPROACHES

Surgical Techniques
- modified Broström—both ligaments are taken off their origin on the fibula and tagged with a retraction suture; the inferior extensor retinaculum is identified and retracted distally; the peroneals are checked for tears and retracted plantarward; a periosteal elevator is used on the distal fibula to lift a flap; the tip of the bone is rasped
- separate suture anchors (3.5-mm bioabsorbable) are inserted at the old origin of the ATF and CF ligaments; these suture anchors are than tied into the foreshortened ligaments with the talus posteriorly translated and in 5° of dorsiflexion and the hindfoot in 5° of eversion
- the inferior retinaculum is pulled proximally and sewn over the ligaments using the same suture and needles; the periosteum is than sutured over the top
- if there is insufficient ligament for an anatomic-type reconstruction, the repair should be augmented prior to placing the suture anchors with a split peroneal tenodesis (modified Evans), which takes the anterior half of the tendon left, attached distally, and freed and reattached proximal to the superior peroneal retinaculum
- a drill hole (3.5 mm) is placed from distal to proximal and posterior; the graft is passed in the same direction, then distal to proximal, then anchored into the calcaneus or back onto itself—after it has been secured, the Broström procedure is then completed

POSTOPERATIVE MANAGEMENT

- same as for CPT code 27695 (Chapter 12)

REHABILITATION

- same as for CPT code 27695

COMPLICATIONS

- recurrent instability

SELECTED REFERENCES

Kelikian AS, Romash MM. Ankle and subtalar instability. In: Kelikian AS, ed. Operative treatment of the foot and ankle. Stamford, CT: Appleton & Lange, 1999:299–320.

Messer TM, Cummins CA, Ahn J, Kelikian AS. Outcome of modified Brostrom procedure for chronic ankle instability using suture anchors. Foot Ankle Int 2000;21:996–1003.

NOTES

_____
_____
_____
_____
_____
_____
_____
_____
_____
_____
_____
_____
_____
_____
_____
_____

ARTHROPLASTY, ANKLE; WITH IMPLANT (TOTAL ANKLE)

CPT code   27702 arthroplasty, ankle; with implant (total ankle)

ICD-9 code   716.97 arthritis, osteoarthritis foot and ankle

INDICATIONS

- posttraumatic arthritis
- inflammatory arthritis
- degenerative arthritis
- relative indication: avascular necrosis with minimal collapse
- hemophilic arthritis

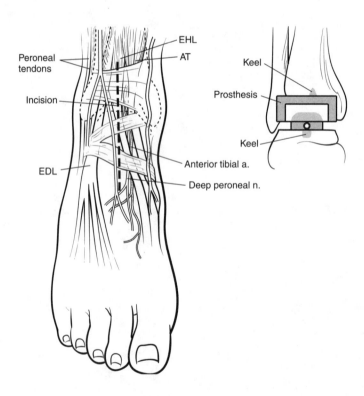

ALTERNATIVE TREATMENTS

- ankle–foot orthosis (AFO)
- Arizona brace
- injections: Hyalgan/Synvisc or corticosteroid
- NSAIDs
- shoe modifications: solid ankle cushion heel (SACH)
- ankle arthrodesis

SURGICAL ANATOMY

Incision

- anterior 15–20 cm length, just lateral to the anterior tibial tendon
- optional lateral incision for the synostosis (tibia-fibula) CPT code 27871

APPROACHES

Surgical Techniques

- a uniplanar external fixator is applied medially with two tibial pins proximal and one talar and one calcaneal 6.5-mm pin distally; the talar pin is placed parallel to the joint surface and any frontal plane deformity is corrected; the ankle is locked in neutral position and distracted 5–10 mm
- the interval between the extensor hallucis longus (EHL) and anterior tibial tendons
- identify the neurovascular bundle, which is just medial and beneath the EHL
- the dorsal branch of the superficial peroneal nerve lies just above the extensor
- incise the retinaculum and preserve the sheath of the anterior tibial tendon
- expose and incise the ankle joint capsule; subperiosteally, with an elevator, expose medially to the malleolus and laterally to the syndesmosis
- rongeur and curette the tibia-fibula syndesmosis
- use a 6-mm burr to prepare the apposing surfaces of the tibia and fibula for a distance of 6 cm above and up to the ankle joint

- the appropriate size (#1–6) tibial cutting block is attached to the jig—determined from preoperative templates; the jig is then lined with the knee and ankle in both the anteroposterior and lateral planes; fine tuning is performed medial/lateral and proximal/distal; verification is performed
- two smooth pins are placed in the jig foot pads (two), then two additional pins are placed into the cutting block
- no more than one-third of the inner surface of the malleoli should be resected; a laminar spreader is placed in the syndesmosis to allow for upsizing and minimizing malleolar resection
- a drill is placed into the medial corner of the cutting block to measure saw depth of the tibia in the sagittal plane and to safeguard from crossing the proximal and medial saw cuts; the proximal (tibial), distal (talar), medial, lateral, and tibial chamfer oscillating saw cuts are completed; the jig and block are removed
- the reciprocating saw is used for the chamfer cut and any retained bone fragments
- the bone removed is then morcellized for later synostosis
- the trial tibial component is inserted
- the fixator is unlocked; then the foot is plantar flexed, and the fixator is re-locked
- the talar cutting guide is positioned from medial to lateral for varus ankle medial and valgus ankle lateral to the midline
- the talar guide is 20° external to the tibial component's spine (external alignment handles)
- a customized router (burr) is used in the talar cutting guide once the trial tibia is removed
- trial reduction of both components is now performed: check in anteroposterior and lateral radiographs, fluoroscopy, and clinical ROM
- the final components are sequentially inserted
- two cancellous 4-mm lag screws are placed for the synostosis into the fibula and tibia percutaneously
- the distal one begins above the tibial fin (keel); overdrill the fibular cortices (3.5 mm) and the tibial cortices to 2.9 mm

- a 4–5 hole, semitubular plate is placed subperiosteally prior to screw insertion, or alternatively, two washers—the second screw is placed 1.5–2 cm proximal to the first (CPT 27871)
- bone graft is placed above the exposed tibial component and between the tib–fib syndesmosis
- final compression is performed; remove the fixator
- the wounds are closed meticulously in interrupted layers
- deflate the tourniquet prior to closure

POSTOPERATIVE MANAGEMENT

- bulky compression dressing with a posterior mold and coaptation splint
- apply short-leg cast at 1 week
- at 3 weeks, remove the cast and sutures
- begin ROM exercises
- at 7 weeks, if the synostosis appears fused, weight-bearing is begun protected with a CAM walker for 4 weeks

COMPLICATIONS

- wound
- intraoperative malleolar fracture
- syndesmotic non-union

SELECTED REFERENCES

Hasselman CT, Wong YS, Conti SF. Total ankle replacement. In: Kitaoka HB, ed. Master techniques in orthopaedic surgery. Philadelphia: Lippincott Williams & Wilkins, 2002:581–595.
Pyevich MT, Alvine FG, Saltzman CL. Total ankle arthroplasty: a unique design. J Bone Joint Surg Am 1998;80A,10:1410–1420.

OSTEOTOMY, TIBIA AND FIBULA

CPT code   **27709 osteotomy, tibia and fibula**

ICD-9 code   **733.81 malunion, fracture**

INDICATIONS

- malunion of distal tibia
- intermediate arthritis of the ankle joint

ALTERNATIVE TREATMENTS

- ankle–foot orthosis (AFO)
- orthotic devices with wedges
- arthrodesis or arthroplasty

SURGICAL ANATOMY

- determine the level and type of deformity
- uni-plane or oblique plane
- magnitude of deformity
- center of rotation of angulation (CORA)

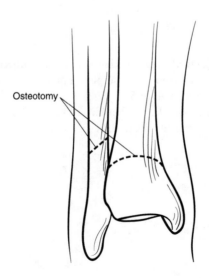

Incision
- depends on location of deformity but usually just lateral to the tibial crest and posterolateral to the fibula

APPROACHES

Surgical Techniques
- longitudinal incision with subperiosteal dissection
- for uniplanar varus/valgus deformity, a dome osteotomy is performed or opened/closed wedge; use multiple drill holes and connect them with an osteotome
- for varus deformity, resect 1 cm of fibula at the level of the tibial osteotomy
- for valgus deformity, perform an oblique osteotomy at the same level
- temporary fixation with a K-wire jail
- final stabilization can be performed with plates, cross screws, staples, uniplanar external fixation, or small-wire circular frame
- the choice of fixation is predicated by the clinical picture and deformity preoperatively

POSTOPERATIVE MANAGEMENT

- predicated by fixation
- with internal fixation splint for 2 weeks followed by cast
- weight bearing with external support at 8–12 weeks
- with external fixation, weight bearing at 6–8 weeks; frame remains on until healed

REHABILITATION

- ROM and strengthening

COMPLICATIONS

- over- or undercorrection
- non-union
- infection
- neuropraxia

SELECTED REFERENCES

Mangone PG. Distal tibial osteotomies for the treatment of foot and ankle disorders. In: Myerson MS, Sammarco GJ, eds. Foot and ankle clinics. Philadelphia: WB Saunders, 2001:583–597.

Paley DP. Ankle malalignment. In: Kelikian AS, ed. Operative treatment of the foot and ankle. Stamford, CT: Appleton & Lange, 1999:547–586.

NOTES

_____
_____
_____
_____
_____
_____
_____
_____
_____
_____

OPEN TREATMENT OF DISTAL TIBIAL FRACTURE, WEIGHT BEARING

CPT code   **27827   open treatment of fracture of the weight-bearing articular surface/portion of distal tibia (e.g., pilon or tibial plafond), with internal or external fixation; of tibia only**

ICD-9 code   **824.8 tibia closed distal end**

INDICATIONS

- comminuted intra-articular fractures of the plafond with displacement

ALTERNATIVE TREATMENTS

- cast
- unilateral frame
- circular frame
- limited open reduction–internal fixation (ORIF) or closed reduction–internal fixation (CRIF)

SURGICAL ANATOMY

- Any of the above options or combinations can be used. Traditionally ORIF with plate fixation has been used. Usually the soft tissue envelope and the fracture pattern dictate the treatment. Initially, some form of temporary or definitive external fixator is applied for the severely comminuted plafond fractures (EBI, Orthofix ankle monolateral frames). A computed tomographic (CT) scan is then recommended to determine the reduction by ligamentotaxis and to allow for the four-quadrant analysis to help decide on the anatomic safe corridors for small-wire or cannulated screw fixation

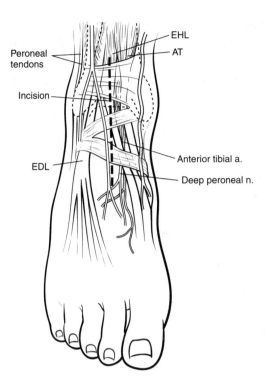

Incision

- limited for use with direct or indirect reduction techniques—unless there is syndesmotic involvement, fibular plating is not necessary

APPROACHES

- incisions are between 4 and 6 cm to avoiding undermining flaps
- the joint surface is disimpacted
- fracture lines in the coronal plane are transfixed with wire from the cannulated 4-mm set
- a decision for either a monolateral frame with percutaneous screw or plate fixation vs. standard use of the circular frame

Surgical Techniques
- with a sterile traction bow in the calcaneus, the proximal ring bloc is transfixed to the tibia with small wires and 5-mm half-pins; the articular fixation and reduction are performed with or without cannulated screws; olive wires can be used for small articular fragments; reduction forceps (AO 916) can also be employed
- the distal ring is then attached as well as a foot frame if needed— the overall goal should be for restoration of length, alignment, and articular restoration, but not at the cost of compromising the soft tissue envelope (which increases the risk of major wound problems) and infection (which would impair future reconstructive procedures—arthrodesis and arthroplasty)

POSTOPERATIVE MANAGEMENT

- non-weight-bearing usually for 3–4 months

REHABILITATION

- ROM and strengthening

COMPLICATIONS

- posttraumatic arthritis, osteomyelitis, wound necrosis, and malalignment

SELECTED REFERENCES

French B, Tornetta P. Hybrid external fixation of tibial pilon fractures.
  In: Thordson DB, Myerson MS, eds. Foot and ankle clinics: the ankle.
  Philadelphia: WB Saunders, 2000:853–871.
Kodros SA. Pilon fractures. In: Kelikian AS, ed. Operative treatment of
  the foot and ankle. Stamford, CT: Appleton & Lange, 1999:285–298.
Watson JT, Tibial pilon fractures. In: Morandi MM, Browner BD, eds.
  Techniques in orthopedics. Hagerstown, MD: Lippincott-Raven,
  1996:150–159.

NOTES

_____
_____
_____
_____
_____
_____
_____
_____
_____
_____
_____
_____
_____
_____
_____

OPEN TREATMENT OF DISTAL TIBIOFIBULAR JOINT DISRUPTION

CPT code   27829 open treatment of distal tibiofibular joint (syndesmosis)
                          disruption, with or without internal or external fixation

ICD-9 codes   845   sprain ligaments
                   824.2 fracture lateral malleolus closed (with syndesmotic ligament
                          disruption)

INDICATIONS

- when stabilizing a displaced fibular fracture, a manual Cotton stress test is done intraoperatively via a Ragnell retractor along the medial border of the fibula and applying lateral traction under direct and fluoroscopic view; if there is medial opening or tibial-fibular widening, then transsyndesmotic stabilization is indicated regardless of the level of fibular fracture (Weber B or C fracture)
- when fibular fixation is not required, i.e., Weber C (high pronation external rotation—PER IV), a manual examination is required
- late reconstruction for chronic tibial-fibular instability

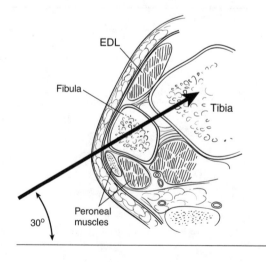

ALTERNATIVE TREATMENTS

- closed techniques, although difficult to attain and maintain reduction criteria

SURGICAL ANATOMY

Incision

- percutaneous along the posterolateral surface of the fibula, 2 cm proximal to the talocrural joint (Weber C high)
- when fibular plating is done, use one of the existing screw holes

APPROACHES

Surgical Techniques

- sandbag under the ipsilateral buttocks
- under fluoroscopic control, overdrill both fibular cortices with a 4.5-mm bit, dropping the drill 30–60° toward the floor (see figure)
- the lateral and medial tibial cortices are drilled with a 2.5-mm bit
- the ankle is held in 0–5° of dorsiflexion
- a large tenaculum can be placed around the medial tibia and lateral fibula to aid the syndesmotic reduction
- after tapping measure with the depth gauge and checking under fluoroscopic control in both planes to verify the screw is intraosseous, a 4.5-mm stainless steel or resorbable screw is inserted; the prominent head may be shaved down with a saw or bipolar cautery if bulky after final positioning
- alternatively, 3.5-mm cortical standard screws using only three cortices fixation or transsyndesmotic staples may be employed

POSTOPERATIVE MANAGEMENT

- non-weight-bearing cast, 6 weeks
- begin active and passive ROM at 6 weeks
- protected weight bearing in a CAM walker from weeks 8–12
- screws are not routinely removed
- sports at 16–20 weeks

COMPLICATIONS

- with standard screw fixation, loosening, breakage, or syndesmotic ossification
- loss of reduction is rare but may occur

SELECTED REFERENCES

Kelikian AS. Ankle fractures. In: Kelikian AS, ed. Operative treatment of the foot and ankle. Stamford, CT: Appleton & Lange, 1999.

NOTES

_____
_____
_____
_____
_____
_____
_____
_____
_____
_____
_____

ARTHRODESIS, ANKLE, ANY METHOD

CPT code   **27870   arthrodesis ankle, any method**

ICD-9 codes   **716.97 arthritis, osteoarthritis, foot and ankle**
                            714   rheumatoid arthritis (RA)

INDICATIONS

- posttraumatic, degenerative, or inflammatory arthritis; avascular necrosis
- failure of nonoperative measures
- neuromuscular deformities

ALTERNATIVE TREATMENTS

- ankle–foot orthosis (AFO)
- rocker-soled shoe, solid ankle cushion heel (SACH)
- nonsteroidal-type drugs
- corticosteroid injections
- Hyalgan/Synvisc injections
- arthroscopic ankle fusion (minor deformities only)
- total ankle arthroplasty (CPT code 27702)

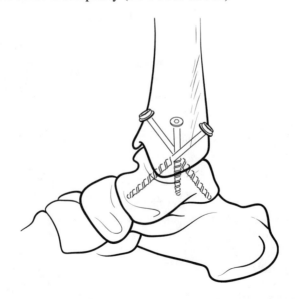

SURGICAL ANATOMY

Incision
- lateral transfibular

APPROACHES

Surgical Techniques
- numerous approaches exist: mini medial and lateral, arthroscopic, posterolateral, and anterior
- fixation: screws, external fixation, blade plate, and locking plate
- fibula is osteotomized 5 cm from its tip, the inner third is resected, and the remainder is reflected posterior in younger patients (otherwise it is entirely removed and morcellized for graft in young patients; the fibula is onlayed back prior to closure for possible conversion to total ankle arthroplasty in future)
- a capsulotomy is performed laterally, and the remaining cartilage is removed
- use a laminar spreader, ring curettes, and a 6-mm burr to decorticate
- the concave tibial and convex talar surfaces are maintained
- realignment is paramount
- the ankle should be positioned in 0–5° dorsiflexion, 5° valgus, and 10° external rotation
- posterior talar displacement will decrease the lever arm of the foot
- guide pins are used from a 7.3-mm or 8.0-mm cannulated system: first is from the posterolateral tibia into the talar neck, second is from medial to lateral at a 45° angle from the tibia to the talus, and third is from the anterolateral tibia to the posterior talus; these are measured and then drilled
- washers are used except medially, large cancellous screws are used, anterolateral screw is 5 to 6.5 mm

POSTOPERATIVE MANAGEMENT

- bulky compression dressing, posterior splint
- sutures are removed at 2 weeks
- short-leg weight-bearing cast at 4 weeks
- CAM walker at 6 weeks

COMPLICATIONS

- non-union, 10%
- malalignment
- ipsilateral distal arthritis

SELECTED REFERENCES

Kelikian AS. Ankle arthrodesis. In: Kelikian AS, ed. Operative treatment of the foot and ankle. Stamford, CT: Appleton & Lange, 1999:351–368.

NOTES

_____
_____
_____
_____
_____
_____
_____
_____
_____
_____
_____

AMPUTATON, LEG, THROUGH TIBIA; WITH IMMEDIATE FITTING TECHNIQUE

CPT code   27881 amputation, leg, through tibia; with immediate fitting technique including application of first cast

ICD-9 codes   443.9   peripheral vascular disease
230.1   osteomyelitis, chronic
733.82 fracture non-union
823.90 fracture tibia, open

INDICATIONS

- peripheral vascular disease with failed bypass or not salvageable
- chronic osteomyelitis
- multiple failed non-union
- nonbraceable Charcot deformity
- type IIIB–C open fracture; unsalvageable limb

ALTERNATIVE TREATMENTS

- limb salvage: vascular, free tissue transfer, or Ilizarov techniques

SURGICAL ANATOMY

Incision

- at the junction of the middle and distal thirds of the leg, between 13 and 18 cm below the knee, a transverse incision is marked spanning two thirds of the anteroposterior diameter of the limb; the medial and lateral posterior longitudinal incisions are of equal length to the transverse one; where they meet proximal, they are curved up proximal to decrease dog ears; distal they meet transverse through the posterior skin

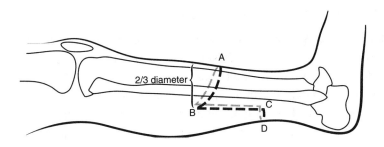

APPROACHES

Surgical Techniques

- the anterior compartment muscles are cut
- the deep and superficial peroneal nerves are cut sharply under tension; then the anterior tibial artery and vein are identified and ligated
- the tibia is transected 1 cm proximal to the anterior skin incision with a Gigli or oscillating saw and then beveled 60° anteriorly
- the fibula is cut 1 cm proximal to the fibula
- the leg is than flexed using a bone hook into the tibial canal
- the deep posterior compartment is divided, then the peroneal and posterior tibial artery and vein are visualized and ligated separately
- a large amputation knife is used to separate the interval between the deep and superficial posterior compartments
- the posterior tibial nerve is cut under tension
- the closure is begun after the tourniquet has been released and bleeding has been controlled
- the posterior fascia is brought forward to the periosteum or anterior tibial drill holes
- the skin and subcutaneous tissue are closed over a drain, which remains for 24 hours

POSTOPERATIVE MANAGEMENT

- non-adherent gauze over the wound followed by 4 × 4 gauze pads, two ABD pads, then a sterile stump sock, and a light layer of cast padding; either an immediate postoperative prosthesis (IPOP) or cast above the knee with a patellar cutout is applied
- when using an IPOP (Air-Limb by Aircast), an inflatable, adjustable shell with turnbuckle straps and air bags inflated between 20 and 30 mm Hg allows for early postoperative weight bearing, 25–30% of body weight

COMPLICATIONS

- wound healing
- phantom and neuroma pain
- tibial-fibular instability (treat with synostosis)

SELECTED REFERENCES

Melamed EA, Schon LC. Lower amputation as a salvage for severe trauma. In: Myerson MS, ed. Foot and ankle clinics. Philadelphia: WB Saunders, 1999:77–96.

Smithy DG. Principles of partial foot amputations in the diabetic. In: Myerson MS, ed. Foot and ankle clinics. Philadelphia: WB Saunders, 1997:171–186.

NOTES

_____

_____

_____

_____

_____

_____

_____

_____

_____

_____

_____

ANKLE DISARTICULATION (SYME'S)

CPT code   27889 ankle disarticulation (Syme's)

ICD-9 code   443.9 peripheral vascular disease (PVD)

INDICATIONS

- patient with an intact heel pad requiring amputation for peripheral vascular disease (PVD), posttraumatic, or congenital deficiencies such as fibular hemimelia, proximal femoral focal deficiency (PFFD), or pseudarthrosis
- when a transmetatarsal amputation is not possible, decrease energy consumption; then do below-the-knee amputation
- adequate perfusion of the heel pad is required

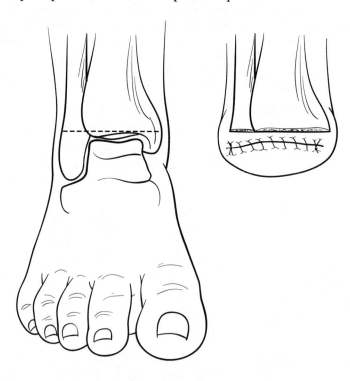

SURGICAL ANATOMY

Incision
- anterior beginning 1 cm distal to each malleoli
- the two starting points are then connected by another incision going in a plantar direction toward the sole of the foot

APPROACHES

Surgical Techniques
- the anterior incision is developed down to the talar dome
- the plantar incision is taken down to the calcaneus; both the medial and lateral ligaments are cut
- a bone hook is placed into the talar dome with distal and plantar traction
- the tarsal tunnel is identified and the neurovascular bundle is protected
- a Key elevator is used to develop a full-thickness skin flap off the calcaneus
- the Achilles is sharply dissected from its heel attachment
- all the anterior tendons are clamped and cut under tension; the anterior tibial artery and veins are ligated
- both malleoli are cut with a saw at the level of the plafond
- the heel pad is brought forward to check the final closure
- multiple drill holes are placed in the distal anterior tibia
- sutures are placed through the drill holes and then the plantar fascia using 0 Vicryl
- the closure is continued over a deep suction drain in an interrupted fashion

POSTOPERATIVE MANAGEMENT
- a posterior mold or short-leg cast is applied
- the cast is changed in 10–14 days
- sutures are removed at 4 weeks
- in non dysvascular patients, weight bearing can begin at 4 weeks
- casting is continued for a total of 6–8 weeks
- a CAM walker may be used until prosthetic fitting at 12 weeks
- a polypropylene AFO with a solid ankle cushion heel (SACH)

COMPLICATIONS

- delayed wound healing
- fat pad migration
- painful neuroma

SELECTED REFERENCES

Brodsky JW. Syme amputation. In: Kitaoko HB, ed. Master techniques in orthopaedic surgery: the foot and ankle. Philadelphia: Lippincott Williams & Wilkins, 2002:615–629.

NOTES

_____
_____
_____
_____
_____
_____
_____
_____
_____
_____
_____

TENOTOMY, PERCUTANEOUS, TOE; SINGLE TENDON

CPT code   28010 tenotomy, percutaneous, toe; single tendon

ICD-9 code   735.4 mallet toe, hammer toe

INDICATIONS

- flexible mallet toe

ALTERNATIVE TREATMENTS

- wide toe-box shoe, crest bars, silicone digital pads
- terminal Syme's amputation
- flexor to extensor transfer
- distal interphalangeal joint fusion

SURGICAL ANATOMY

- relationship between the digital neurovascular bundles and the flexor hallucis longus (FHL) tendon

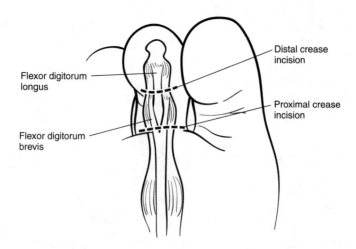

Incision
- transverse at the distal toe flexion crease

APPROACHES

Surgical Techniques
- linear spreading with medial and lateral retraction
- tenotomy of desired tendon done at either distal or proximal level

POSTOPERATIVE MANAGEMENT

- extension splinting for 3 weeks

REHABILITATION

toe extension exercises

COMPLICATIONS

- recurrence

SELECTED REFERENCES

Murphy GA. Mallet toe deformity. In: Richardson GE, Myerson MS, eds. Foot and ankle clinics: lesser toe deformities. Philadelphia: WB Saunders, 1998:279–292.

NOTES

_____
_____
_____
_____
_____
_____
_____
_____
_____
_____
_____

TARSAL TUNNEL RELEASE

CPT code   **28035 release tarsal tunnel (posterior tibial nerve)**

ICD-9 code   **355.5 tarsal tunnel syndrome**

INDICATIONS

- symptomatic patient with posteromedial pain
- positive Tinel's sign, sensory deficit (Semmes-Weinstein monofilaments, 5.07)
- positive compression test with ankle dorsiflexion and hindfoot eversion
- abductor digiti minimi weakness
- electromyography (EMG) and nerve conduction velocity (NCV) studies to rule out a proximal or other lesion (25% of true tarsal tunnel syndrome have negative study)
- to rule out space-occupying lesion in tarsal tunnel via MRI or ultrasonography
- failure to respond to nonoperative treatment modalities

ALTERNATIVE TREATMENTS

- NSAIDs, iontophoresis, corticosteroid injection
- orthotic devices

SURGICAL ANATOMY

Incision
- the posterior tibial nerve, first branch is the calcaneal
- the medial and lateral branches bifurcate at the midportion of the malleolar calcaneal axis
- the lateral plantar nerve gives off a branch to the abductor digiti minimi muscle (Baxter's nerve) beneath the deep abductor hallucis fascia
- "To Destroy Vengeance Allow No Hatred," a mnemonic for anatomic structures from anterior to posterior: PT (posterior tibial tendon), FDL, Vein, Artery, Nerve, FHL

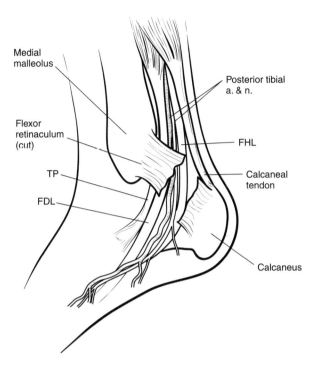

Medial malleolus

Flexor retinaculum (cut)

TP

FDL

Posterior tibial a. & n.

FHL

Calcaneal tendon

Calcaneus

APPROACHES

Surgical Techniques

- 8–10 cm incision along the course of the posterior tibial nerve
- blunt dissection to avoid undermining skin flaps
- identify the vein, artery, and nerve proximally in the wound after cutting the flexor retinaculum
- trace the nerve distally to its main bifurcation
- release the tarsal tunnel distal (i.e., beneath the abductor hallucis) by incising the superficial and deep fascia (retract the muscle distally and plantarward)
- check for any soft tissue masses in the tunnel
- deflate the tourniquet and obtain meticulous hemostasis
- closure is superficial and skin only

POSTOPERATIVE MANAGEMENT

- splint for 10–14 days, non-weight-bearing
- sutures for 21 days

SELECTED REFERENCES

Kodros SA. Nerve entrapment. In: Kelikian AS, ed. Operative treatment
    of the foot and ankle. Stamford, CT: Appleton & Lange, 1999:201–210.
Ballie D, Kelikian AS. Tarsal tunnel syndrome. Foot Ankle Int 1998;19:65.

NOTES

EXCISION OF MORTON'S NEUROMA

CPT code   **28080 excision, interdigital (Morton) neuroma, single, each**

ICD-9 code   **355.6 neuroma**

INDICATIONS

- symptomatic interdigital pain at the third and fourth web space (90%) or second and third web space (10%)
- rule out other causes of metatarsalgia including the second intermetatarsal space syndrome
- failed nonoperative measures which include shoe wear, medications, metatarsal pads, and corticosteroid injections
- ultrasonography is an excellent diagnostic tool for equivocal cases

ALTERNATIVE TREATMENTS

- as described in indications above
- intermetatarsal ligament release alone if minimal involvement

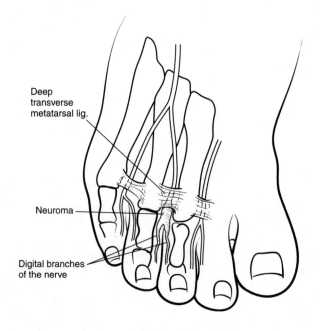

Deep transverse metatarsal lig.

Neuroma

Digital branches of the nerve

SURGICAL ANATOMY

- both web spaces, 1–3%
- bilateral, 15%

Incision
- 3–4 cm in dorsal web space
- if exploring both web spaces, place incision over third metatarsal

Surgical Techniques
- dissect to the deep transverse intermetatarsal ligament
- place a right angle Mixter forceps underneath the ligament and release it completely
- a tonsillar retractor or small laminar spreader is placed between the metatarsal shafts
- if excision is to be performed, cut distal digital branches first
- the distal ends are clamped and all plantar branches are freed
- the nerve is traced 2–3 cm proximal to the neuroma
- the medial and lateral trunks are visualized for 3–4 web space
- with distal traction the nerve is cut as far proximal as possible

POSTOPERATIVE MANAGEMENT

- postoperative shoe
- sutures out at 3 weeks
- encourage toe flexion exercises

COMPLICATIONS

- recurrence
- stump neuroma
- delayed wound healing

SELECTED REFERENCES

Hort KR, DeOrio JK. Adjacent interdigital nerve irritation: single incision surgical treatment. Foot Ankle Int 2002;23:1026–1030.
Kodros SA. Nerve entrapment. In: Kelikian AS, ed. Operative treatment of the foot & ankle. Stamford, CT: Appleton & Lange, 1999:201–210.

EXCISION OF LESION, TENDON, TENDON SHEATH, OR CAPSULE; FOOT

CPT code   **28090** excision of lesion, tendon, tendon sheath, or capsule
(including synovectomy) (e.g., cyst or ganglion); foot

ICD-9 code   **727.42** ganglion of tendon sheath

INDICATIONS

• rare, only if causing pain with shoe wear

ALTERNATIVE TREATMENTS

• aspiration with or without corticosteroid injection

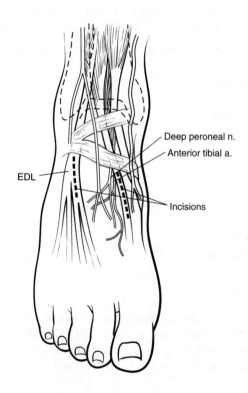

SURGICAL ANATOMY

- in the foot, dorsal neuromas (incisional) are common

Incision
- linear

APPROACHES

Surgical Techniques
- careful dissection to the joint or tendon; the stalk must be removed as well

POSTOPERATIVE MANAGEMENT

- compression dressing with suture removal at 2 weeks

REHABILITATION

- ROM toes

COMPLICATIONS

- recurrence high
- incisional neuromas

SELECTED REFERENCES

Giannestras NJ. Foot disorders, 2nd ed. London: Lea & Febiger, 1973: 612–613.

NOTES

_____
_____
_____
_____
_____
_____
_____
_____

OSTECTOMY, COMPLETE EXCISION; ALL METATARSAL HEADS, EXCLUDING FIRST METATARSAL HEAD

CPT code   28114 ostectomy, complete excision; all metatarsal heads, with partial proximal phalangectomy, excluding 1st metatarsal head (e.g., Clayton-type procedure)

ICD-9 code   714   rheumatoid arthritis
                  726.70 metatarsalgia

INDICATIONS

- painful plantar callosities with joint destruction
- rheumatoid forefoot with MTP subluxation

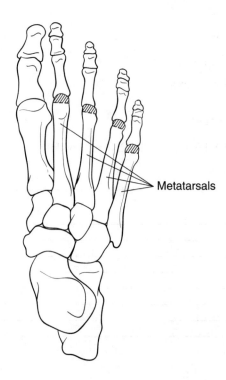

Metatarsals

ALTERNATIVE TREATMENTS

- metatarsal pads or bars, extra-depth shoes, orthotic devices
- metatarsal osteotomies (e.g., Weil, CPT code 28308)
- condylectomy (CPT code 28288)

SURGICAL ANATOMY

- the lateral and dorsal subluxation of the lesser toes combined with proliferative synovitis (rheumatoid arthritis) augments the deformity and pressure plantarward

Incision
- dorsal web-splitting incisions between the second and third toes and the fourth and fifth toes, about 4–5 cm in length

APPROACHES

- the plantar approach just distal to the metatarsal heads can also be used but is more extensive

Surgical Techniques
- the extensor mechanism is retracted and the metatarsal neck is exposed; the head is resected at the neck with the saw blade directed proximal and plantar
- a McGlamry retractor is placed under the metatarsal head prior; once the resection has been completed, the capital fragment is grasped with a towel clip axially and gently stripped by a clockwise and counter clockwise motion of its soft tissue attachments—the same is done for the remaining lesser metatarsals
- at this point, if the toe deformity is still present one can attempt a closed osteoclasis at the proximal interphalangeal joint
- otherwise a partial proximal phalangectomy is performed by extending the incision along the toes in the mid-axial line
- the proximal third is resected; if the toes are floppy, a syndactylization is performed between the adjacent toes

POSTOPERATIVE MANAGEMENT

- bulky compression dressing with suture removal at 3 weeks

REHABILITATION

- ROM toes

COMPLICATIONS

- recurrence

SELECTED REFERENCES

Kelikian AS. Rheumatoid arthritis of the foot and ankle. In: Kelikian AS, ed. Operative treatment of the foot and ankle. Stamford, CT: Appleton & Lange 1999:179–199.
Kelikian H, Clayton L, Loseff H. Surgical syndactylia of the toes. Clin Orthop 1961;19:208.

NOTES

_____
_____
_____
_____
_____
_____
_____
_____
_____
_____
_____
_____
_____
_____

OSTECTOMY, EXCISION OF TARSAL COALITION

CPT code   28116 ostectomy, excision of tarsal coalition

ICD-9 code   755.67 tarsal coalition

INDICATIONS

- symptomatic tarsal coalition without arthritis, not responsive to conservative treatment

ALTERNATIVE TREATMENTS

- short-leg weight-bearing cast, UCBL orthotic device
- arthrodesis—subtalar versus triple

SURGICAL ANATOMY

- 1% of the population has a coalition. Calcaneonavicular and talonavicular are the two most common. There should be no superimposed arthritis of the transverse tarsal or subtalar joints. A coalition of the talocalcaneal joint should be <25%

Incision
- for calcaneonavicular bars, a sinus tarsi (Ollier) incision is made in Langer's skin lines
- for talocalcaneal (middle facet) bars, an incision is made centered over the sustentaculum tali just below the posterior tibial tendon

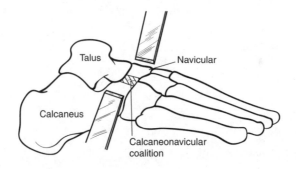

APPROACHES

- the calcaneonavicular bar is exposed after reflecting the extensor digitorum brevis (EDB) distally; the talonavicular joint is exposed and protected
- a trapezoidal segment of bone is removed using two, 12-mm-wide osteotomes, which converge, from the talonavicular and calcaneonavicular joints
- after the bar been removed, there should be a 12-mm space and nearly full supination and pronation; the EDB is interposed in the space

Surgical Techniques

- talocalcaneal bars are more difficult; the posterior tibial tendon is reflected dorsally, whereas the flexor digitorum longus (FDL) and flexor hallucis longus (FHL) are retracted plantarward—fluoroscopic identification of the bar and its margins is critical in the lateral and axial planes
- at this point, osteotomes are inserted above and below the bar, which is then carefully resected; split FDL tendon or free gluteal fat may be interposed; one should ensure there is full hindfoot and forefoot motion

POSTOPERATIVE MANAGEMENT

- splint in inversion and supination
- begin ROM at 2 weeks
- protected weight bearing (CAM walker) at 4 weeks

REHABILITATION

- passive ROM and active-assisted ROM

COMPLICATIONS

- recurrence of bar

SELECTED REFERENCES

Mosier KM, Asher M. Tarsal coalition and peroneal spastic flatfoot: a review. J Bone Joint Surg Am 1984;66:976.
Quill GE. Subtalar joint reconstruction. In: Kelikian AS, ed. Operative treatment of the foot and ankle. Stamford, CT: Appleton & Lange, 1999:433–454.

NOTES

_____

_____

_____

_____

_____

_____

_____

_____

_____

_____

OSTECTOMY, CALCANEUS

CPT code   28118 ostectomy, calcaneus

ICD-9 code   726.71 Achilles tendonitis, retrocalcaneal bursitis (Haglund's deformity)

INDICATIONS

• posterior heel pain with an increased Fowler/Phillip angle that does not respond to nonoperative measures

ALTERNATIVE TREATMENTS

• backless shoes, Silo socks, heel stretches, trial of casting
• rule out associated tendon pathology with ultrasonography or MRI

SURGICAL ANATOMY

• determine if the pain is posterolateral, posteromedial, or both

Incision
• based on area of maximal tenderness and x-ray markers (lateral and axial)

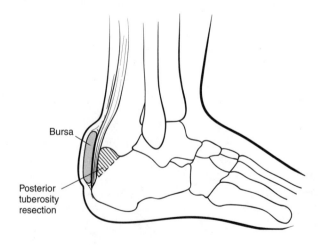

APPROACHES

- if lateral approach, place the patient in the decubitus position with affected side up
- if medial, extended inverted L, or combined approach, have the patient prone

Surgical Techniques
- the medial or lateral incisions are 1.5 cm anterior to the Achilles tendon and carried down to the retrocalcaneal bursae; avoid the sural nerve lateral and the medial calcaneal nerve; the bursae are resected and the Achilles fibers retracted posteriorly
- an osteotome is inserted 1 cm anterior to the superior angle of the calcaneus and extended posterior to the level of the Achilles insertion
- if there is insertional calcification, which appears to be the major clinical problem, a transverse incision, 4 cm in length distally, at the junction of the ankle and heel crease beginning at the distal aspect of the medial incision
- the tendon is reattached via drill holes (no. 2 FiberWire) and/or suture anchors

POSTOPERATIVE MANAGEMENT

- for simple excisions, a posterior splint for 10–14 days followed by a CAM walker for 2 weeks
- for reattachments, the protocol is similar to secondary Achilles repair (CPT code 27654)

REHABILITATION

- ROM at 2 weeks

COMPLICATIONS

- recurrent pain, 10–15%

SELECTED REFERENCES

Digiovanni BF, Gould JS. Achilles tendonitis and posterior heel disorders.
   In: Myerson MS, ed. Foot and ankle clinics: contemporary approach to
   the Achilles tendon. Philadelphia: WB Saunders, 1997:411–428.
Wapner KL. Achilles tendon ruptures and posterior heel pain. In: Kelikian
   AS, ed. Operative treatment of the foot and ankle. Stamford, CT:
   Appleton & Lange, 1999:369–387.

NOTES

_____
_____
_____
_____
_____
_____
_____
_____
_____
_____
_____

TALECTOMY, ASTRAGALECTOMY

CPT code   28130 talectomy (astragalectomy)

ICD-9 code   754.70 clubfoot

INDICATIONS

- recurrent rigid clubfoot (arthrogryposis)
- type IV—open talus fracture/dislocation
- chronic osteomyelitis

ALTERNATIVE TREATMENTS

- Ilizarov with correction

SURGICAL ANATOMY

- the talus is devoid of any motor attachments—only ligaments and capsule

Incision
- anterior longitudinal (CPT code 27625)

APPROACHES

Surgical Techniques
- the talus is extracted after sectioning its medial and lateral ligament attachments; if the head and neck fragment can be retained there is less dissociation of the Chopart joint
- in clean, skeletally mature cases, a tibiocalcaneal fusion can be performed (CPT code 28705); otherwise an axial, large 3.5-mm K-wire can be placed in the heel retrograde for temporary stabilization

POSTOPERATIVE MANAGEMENT

- cast non-weight-bearing for 4 weeks, followed by walking cast

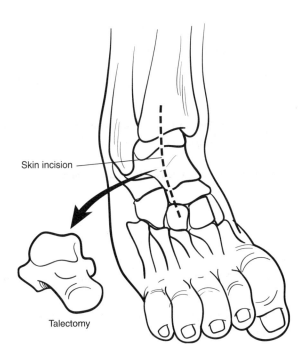

Skin incision

Talectomy

REHABILITATION

- gait training, rocker bottom shoe, and 2-cm heel-sole lift

COMPLICATIONS

- leg length discrepancy

SELECTED REFERENCES

Kelikian H, Kelikian AS. Disorders of the ankle. Philadelphia: WB
  Saunders, 1984:706–716.

NOTES

_____
_____
_____
_____
_____
_____

REPAIR, TENDON, FLEXOR, FOOT; PRIMARY OR SECONDARY, WITHOUT FREE GRAFT, EACH TENDON

CPT code   28200 repair, tendon, flexor, foot; primary or secondary, without free
                  graft, each tendon

ICD-9 code   893.2 open wound of toes with tendon involvement

INDICATIONS

- if there is nerve involvement as well, then exploration and repair are indicated
- for isolated flexor hallucis longus (FHL) tendon laceration, controversy exists
- if both the FHL and flexor digitorum brevis (FDB) of the great toe are lacerated then repair is indicated

ALTERNATIVE TREATMENTS

- nonoperative treatment does provide good functional outcomes

SURGICAL ANATOMY

Incision
- most repairs can be done through the original open incision, which can be extended proximally or distally if needed

APPROACHES

Surgical Techniques
- Kessler- or Bunnell-type suture technique with a 2–0 nonabsorbable suture

POSTOPERATIVE MANAGEMENT

- short-leg non-weight-bearing cast with a distal extension to block toe extension in 10° equinus for 4 weeks, followed by short-leg weight-bearing cast for 2 weeks

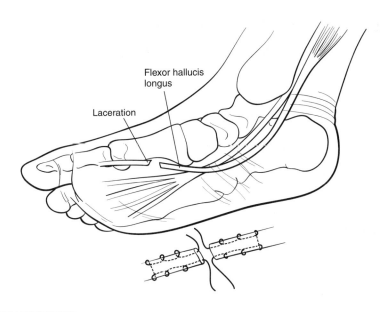

REHABILITATION

- passive toe flexion at 2 weeks, and active exercises at 6 weeks

COMPLICATIONS

- 39% have loss of restoration of toe flexion

SELECTED REFERENCES

Scaduto AA, Cracchiolo A. Lacerations and ruptures of the flexor or extensor hallucis longus tendons. In: Cracchiolo A, Myerson MS. Foot and ankle clinics: the hallux. Philadelphia: WB Saunders, 2000:725–736.

NOTES

_____
_____
_____
_____
_____
_____
_____
_____
_____

REPAIR, TENDON, EXTENSOR, FOOT; PRIMARY OR SECONDARY, EACH TENDON

CPT code   **28208 repair, tendon, extensor, foot; primary or secondary, each tendon**

ICD-9 code   **893.2 open wound of toes with tendon laceration**

INDICATIONS

- indicated in most cases
- spontaneous rupture is rare

ALTERNATIVE TREATMENTS

- late MTP fusion

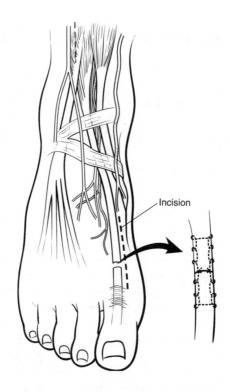

Incision

SURGICAL ANATOMY

- extensor digitorum brevis (EDB) lies just lateral to the extensor hallucis longus (EHL) tendon

Incision

- laceration wound may be extended proximally and distally as needed

APPROACHES

Surgical Techniques

- 3–0 nonabsorbable suture is used with a Kessler, Bunnell, or Krackow technique

POSTOPERATIVE MANAGEMENT

- short-leg cast with flexion block 6 weeks

REHABILITATION

- passive toe extension at 3 weeks

COMPLICATIONS

- adhesions

SELECTED REFERENCES

Scaduto AA, Cracchiolo A. Lacerations and ruptures of the flexor or extensor hallucis longus tendons. In: Cracchiolo A, Myerson MS, eds. Foot and ankle clinics: the hallux. Philadelphia: WB Saunders, 2000: 725–736.

CAPSULOTOMY PROCEDURE

CPT code   **28270 capsulotomy; metatarsophalangeal joint, with or without tenorrhaphy, each joint (separate procedure)**

ICD-9 code   **735.5 claw toe acquired**

INDICATIONS

- not responsive to nonoperative modalities

ALTERNATIVE TREATMENTS

- wide toe-box shoe, cross-tapping of the toe, Budin pads
- metatarsal shortening osteotomies (Weil, CPT code 28308)
- flexor to extensor transfer (CPT code 27690)

SURGICAL ANATOMY

Incision
- dorsal linear

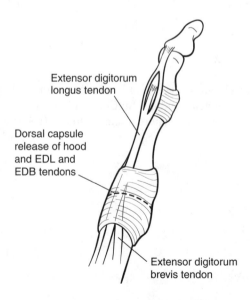

Extensor digitorum longus tendon

Dorsal capsule release of hood and EDL and EDB tendons

Extensor digitorum brevis tendon

APPROACHES

Surgical Techniques

- sequentially the MTP capsule, and longus and brevis tendons are sectioned; if needed, the collateral ligaments are also released

POSTOPERATIVE MANAGEMENT

- extension block splint

REHABILITATION

- toe, passive flexion exercises

COMPLICATIONS

- recurrence

SELECTED REFERENCES

Sands AK, Byck DC. Idiopathic clawed toes. In: Richardson GE, Myerson MS, eds. Foot and ankle clinics: lesser toe deformities. Philadelphia: WB Saunders, 1998:245–258.

NOTES

_____
_____
_____
_____
_____
_____
_____
_____
_____
_____

SYNDACTYLIZATION, TOES

CPT code   28280 syndactylization, toes (e.g., webbing or Kelikian-type procedure)

ICD-9 codes   700   clavus (corns/callus)
                   735.4 claw toes

INDICATIONS

- intractable interdigital soft corns
- dislocated claw toe
- floppy toe (post phalangectomy)

ALTERNATIVE TREATMENTS

- trimming and lamb's wool or interdigital pads
- partial condylectomy
- Budin pads for claw toe
- Hoffman procedure with osteoclasis, lesser toe or proximal interphalangeal fusion

SURGICAL ANATOMY

Incision
- web-splitting incision with removal of equal triangular flaps on the adjacent toes

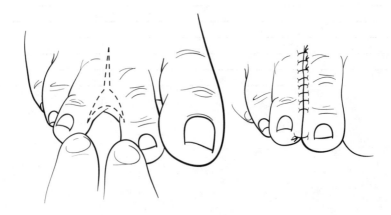

APPROACHES

Surgical Techniques

- dorsal aspect of the triangular flap should begin below the mid-axial line in the sagittal plane
- the partial phalangectomy is either from the base or head of the proximal phalanx, depending on the offending bony prominence
- the extensor and flexor tendons are retracted and protected after subperiosteal dissection
- one-third of the affected portion of the phalanx is osteotomized and removed
- the skin closure begins at the plantar surface in the middle using 3–0 Vicryl and an inverting stitch (inside-out to outside-in)
- equal bites are taken on each side, starting in the center and advancing to the periphery to the tips of each digit
- a 2–0 Vicryl stitch is placed from the tip of one toe to the tip of the other (outside-in to inside-out)
- the dorsal skin is closed from distal to proximal with 3–0 Vicryl, again in an inverted fashion
- the final two proximal sutures are with a 4–0 nylon simple stitch

POSTOPERATIVE MANAGEMENT

- nylon sutures removed at 2 weeks
- syndactilized toes are taped together for 4 weeks

COMPLICATIONS

- weak or floppy toes

SELECTED REFERENCE

Kelikian H. Deformities of the lesser toes. In: Kelikian H. Hallux valgus and allied deformities of the forefoot and metatarsalgia. Philadelphia: WB Saunders, 1965:382–387.

CORRECTION OF HAMMER TOE

CPT code   28285 correction, hammer toe (e.g., interphalangeal fusion, partial or
                    total phalangectomy)

ICD-9 code   735.4 hammer toes

INDICATIONS

* fixed deformity: flexion or clinodactyly at proximal
  interphalangeal or distal interphalangeal (mallet toe) joint

ALTERNATIVE TREATMENTS

* accommodative shoe wear
* toe guards
* toe crest bars (flexible deformity)
* amputation: for revision or elderly
* tendon transfer for flexible deformity (Girdlestone-Taylor)

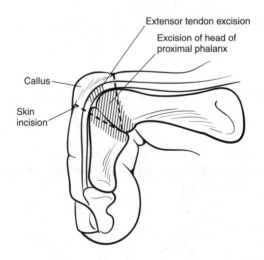

SURGICAL ANATOMY

Incision
- transverse at proximal interphalangeal or digital interphalangeal joint (elliptical at joint if redundancy)
- longitudinal
- T with short limb at distal interphalangeal joint, long limb proximal

APPROACHES

Surgical Techniques
- cut tendon, capsule, collateral ligaments
- remove 3–4 mm of distal portion of proximal phalanx and 1–2 mm of middle phalanx
- place 1.6-mm K-wire antegrade then retrograde across toe
- alternatively, perform only the proximal phalanx cut for a proximal interphalangeal resection arthroplasty
- alternative fusion fixation with an FRS (Foot Reconstruction Set, Ace-DePuy) internal pin
- for claw toes, a metatarsophalangeal capsular and tendon release (CPT code 28270) and or a Weil osteotomy (CPT code 28308)

POSTOPERATIVE MANAGEMENT

- if K-wire is used, remove it at 3 weeks
- tape to adjoining toe for 3 weeks more
- toe flexion exercises at metatarsophalangeal joint
- stiff-soled postoperative shoe, 4 weeks

COMPLICATIONS

- recurrent deformity
- chronic swelling

SELECTED REFERENCES

Sarrafian SK. Correction of fixed hammertoe deformities with resection of the heads of the proximal phalanx and extensor tendon tenodesis. Foot Ankle Int 1995;16:449–451.

Watson AD, Anderson RB, Davis WH. Toe deformities. In: Kelikian AS, ed. Operative treatment of the foot and ankle. Stamford, CT: Appleton & Lange, 1999:99–115.

NOTES

_____
_____
_____
_____
_____
_____
_____
_____
_____
_____
_____

OSTEOTOMY, PARTIAL, EACH METATARSAL HEAD

CPT code   **28288** ostectomy, partial, exostectomy or condylectomy, metatarsal head, each metatarsal head (DuVries condylectomy)

ICD-9 code   **726.70** metatarsalgia

INDICATIONS

- metatarsal transfer lesion of the lesser metatarsals

ALTERNATIVE TREATMENTS

- metatarsal pads, bars, or orthotic devices
- Weil osteotomy (CPT code 28308)

SURGICAL ANATOMY

Incision
- dorsal between the adjacent metatarsals
- if single metatarsal, avoid crossing the extensor crease (curve or Z flap)

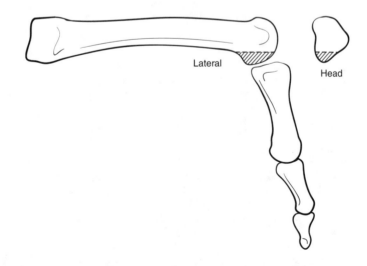

Lateral

Head

APPROACHES

Surgical Techniques
- retract extensor mechanism
- incise dorsal capsule
- place a McGlamry retractor (skid) underneath the metatarsal head
- with a microsagittal saw resect the plantar 25–30% of the head
- use a fine rasp on the undersurface

POSTOPERATIVE MANAGEMENT

- emphasize toe plantar flexion exercises

COMPLICATIONS

- recurrence and transfer lesion

SELECTED REFERENCES

Watson A, Anderson R, Davis H. Metatarsalgia. In: Kelikian AS, ed. Operative treatment of the foot and ankle. Stamford, CT: Appleton & Lange, 1999.

NOTES

_____
_____
_____
_____
_____
_____
_____
_____
_____
_____

CORRECTION OF HALLUX RIGIDUS

CPT code   **28289 hallux rigidus correction with cheilectomy, debridement, and**
                    capsular release of the first metatarsophalangeal joint

ICD-9 code   **735.2 hallux rigidus**

INDICATIONS

- painful hallux rigidus stage I–II, not responsive to conservative measures

ALTERNATIVE TREATMENTS

- stiff-soled shoe with a soft upper last
- carbon fiber orthotic device with a Mortonís extension
- cheilectomy with metatarsal or phalangeal osteotomy

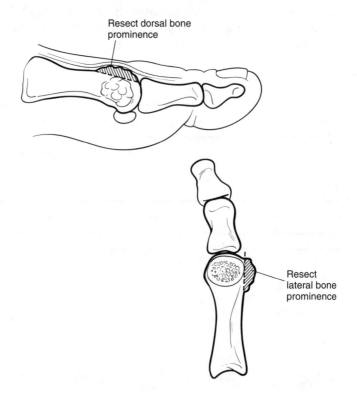

Resect dorsal bone prominence

Resect lateral bone prominence

SURGICAL ANATOMY

Incision
- dorsal, just medial to the extensor hallucis longus (EHL) tendon centered over the metatarsal phalangeal joint
- medial

APPROACHES

Surgical Techniques
- after capsular incision the dorsal surface is exposed
- all osteophytes are removed from the proximal phalanx and medial/lateral metatarsal head
- remove the dorsal 30% of the metatarsal head and rasp the edges
- if >30% of the articular surface is eroded, then metatarsophalangeal fusion is indicated
- the role of concomitant osteotomy remains controversial (Moberg or Weil)
- use a McGlamry retractor or Freer elevator to sesamoidal and capsular adhesions
- one should obtain 70 degrees of dorsiflexion relative to the sole of the foot

POSTOPERATIVE MANAGEMENT

- stiff-soled postoperative shoe for 4 weeks
- begin active and passive dorsiflexion exercises for 10 minutes, three times per day
- sports at 8 weeks

COMPLICATIONS

- instability from overzealous resection
- persistent pain

SELECTED REFERENCES

Haddad S. Hallux rigidus. In: Kelikian AS, ed. Operative treatment of the foot and ankle. Stamford, CT: Appleton & Lange, 1999.

CORRECTION OF HALLUX VALGUS (BUNION)

CPT code   **28290 correction of hallux valgus (bunion), with or without
                 sesamoidectomy; simple exostectomy (e.g., Silver-
                 type procedure)**

ICD-9 code   **735.0 hallux valgus**

INDICATIONS

- painful hallux valgus, not responsive to conservative measures
- as an isolated procedure for an intermetatarsal angle <10°
- as an ancillary procedure in combination with first metatarsal osteotomy

ALTERNATIVE TREATMENTS

- wide toe-box shoe with a soft upper last and a low heel
- ring and ball device to stretch the contact area of the bunion on the shoe
- bunion pads

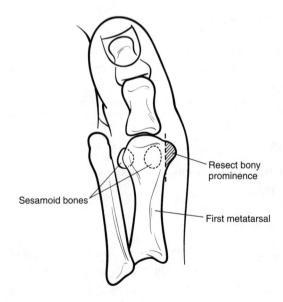

Sesamoid bones

Resect bony prominence

First metatarsal

SURGICAL ANATOMY

Incision
- longitudinal, centered over the medial eminence, 5-cm length

APPROACHES

Surgical Techniques
- the subcutaneous flaps are elevated dorsal and plantar, being careful to identify the dorsomedial cutaneous nerve
- an L-shaped capsulotomy is performed
- alternatively, an elliptical football-shaped portion of capsule is excised
- the medial eminence is exposed
- beginning just medial to the sagittal groove, the eminence is resected with a microsagittal saw from distal to proximal and parallel to the medial border of the foot and not to the first metatarsal shaft
- an adductor tenotomy and lateral capsular release is done with a banana blade via the intra-articular method, from medial to lateral
- after placing the hallux in 5° of varus, the redundant capsule is removed from both limbs of the L (unless the football capsulotomy is used)
- 2–0 Vicryl interrupted sutures are placed

POSTOPERATIVE MANAGEMENT

- a bulky bunion compression dressing is applied
- this is changed to a lighter one at 1 week
- sutures are removed at 2 weeks and a Velcro Jacoby splint is applied
- passive extension exercises are done for 10 minutes
- a stiff-soled postoperative shoe is used for 4 weeks
- at 4 weeks, toe spacers are used and the Jacoby splint is used at night only for 4 weeks more
- sports are permitted at 8 weeks

COMPLICATIONS

- recurrent deformity
- incisional neuroma
- hallux varus

SELECTED REFERENCE

Kelikian AS. Hallux valgus and metatarsus primus varus. In: Kelikian AS, ed. Operative treatment of the foot and ankle. Stamford, CT: Appleton & Lange, 1999.

NOTES

_____
_____
_____
_____
_____
_____
_____
_____
_____
_____

CORRECTION OF HALLUX VALGUS (BUNION) WITH METATARSAL OSTEOTOMY

CPT code   **28296 correction of hallux valgus (bunion), with or without sesamoidectomy; with metatarsal osteotomy (Chevron)**

ICD-9 code   **735.0 hallux valgus—acquired**

INDICATIONS

- painful bunion deformity with intermetatarsal angle <15°, not responsive to shoe-wear modifications

ALTERNATIVE TREATMENTS

- shoe-wear modifications—bunion last

SURGICAL ANATOMY

- the dorsal cutaneous nerve lies dorsomedial

Incision
- medial, 4 cm in length

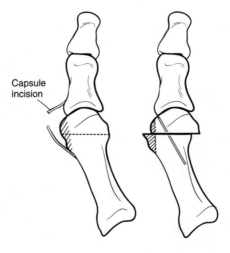

Capsule incision

APPROACHES

- the adductor tenotomy can be performed via the intracapsular method using a no. 67 banana blade; the lateral release can also be performed with a dorsal web-splitting
- incision between the first and second toes

Surgical Techniques

- after the skin has been retracted, the dorsal nerve is protected
- an elliptical portion of medial capsule is excised
- the medial eminence is removed with an oscillating saw starting medial to the medial sagittal saw, avoiding notching of the cortex
- an apex 1 cm distal to the joint is marked; the plantar cut is slightly horizontal and the dorsal cut subtends an angle of 70° to the plantar cut
- the capital fragment is translated 4–5 mm laterally
- a 1.2-mm K-wire is placed from proximal to distal to hold the reduction
- using an antegrade technique, a 1.6-mm K-wire is placed just proximal to dorsal cut through the capital fragment and aiming plantarward
- this is replaced with a bioabsorbable stainless steel 1.5-mm pin, usually between 20 and 25 mm in length
- after the temporary 1.2-mm wire is removed, the resultant stepoff is removed with the saw
- the capsule is closed in a shoelace method using a double armed 3–0 (Maxon) suture

POSTOPERATIVE MANAGEMENT

- a bulky compression dressing with the great toe splinted in neutral varus is applied and changed at 1 week postoperatively
- a Velcro bunion splint is applied at 2 weeks postoperatively and sutures are removed

REHABILITATION

- passive toe extension exercises are encouraged
- the toe is splinted for 4 weeks full time and then 4 weeks nighttime only
- a toe spacer is applied at 4 weeks and a canvas-type shoe wear is allowed

COMPLICATIONS

- recurrence, avascular necrosis (< 5%)

SELECTED REFERENCES

Kelikian AS. Hallux valgus metatarsus primus varus. In: Kelikian AS, ed. Operative treatment of the foot and ankle. Stamford, CT: Appleton & Lange, 1999:61–93.

NOTES

_____
_____
_____
_____
_____
_____
_____
_____
_____
_____

LAPIDUS-TYPE PROCEDURE

CPT code   **28297 Lapidus-type procedure**

ICD-9 code   **735.0 hallux valgus**

INDICATIONS

- hallux valgus metatarsus primus varus intermetatarsal angle >15° and hypermobility of the first ray
- arthritis of the first tarsometatarsal joint
- revision bunion surgery
- contraindicated for short first ray, mild deformity, skeletal immaturity, elderly

ALTERNATIVE TREATMENTS

- see CPT code 28290
- proximal Chevron or dome
- scarf or double osteotomy

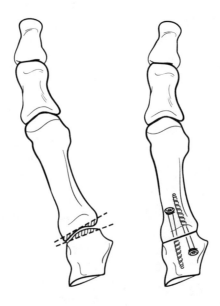

SURGICAL ANATOMY

Incision
- see CPT code 28290
- 5 cm medial to the extensor hallucis longus (EHL) tendon, centered over the first tarsometatarsal joint; beware of the medial dorsocutaneous nerve

APPROACHES

Surgical Techniques
- expose the first tarsometatarsal and protect the anterior tibial and EHL tendons
- a biplanar minimal resection based lateral plantar
- use a long microsagittal saw blade
- a flat small laminar spreader allows deep visualization
- the first metatarsal is plantar flexed, abducted, and supinated (triplanar)
- K-wires from the 4.0-mm cannulated tray are used
- one wire is inserted from proximal to distal and from dorsal to plantar
- the retrograde wire is placed from distal to proximal and from dorsal to plantar—it should be aimed toward the medial aspect of the first cuneiform
- check position and correction with the fluoroscope
- measure, drill (2.9 mm), and countersink
- cannulated cancellous, solid cancellous, or cortical screws (over-drill proximal cortex) may be used
- use leftover bone chips to fill any voids (stress-relieving graft)

POSTOPERATIVE MANAGEMENT

- compression dressing and posterior splint for 2 weeks, then short-leg weight-bearing cast for 4 weeks
- at 6 weeks, postoperative wooden shoe and toe spacer and Jacoby night splint for 4 weeks more
- sports at 12 weeks

COMPLICATIONS

- recurrence rare
- avascular necrosis rare
- shortening, 4–5 mm
- delayed union and non-union, 10%

SELECTED REFERENCES

Kelikian AS. Hallux valgus metatarsus primus varus. In: Kelikian AS, ed. Operative treatment of the foot and ankle. Stamford, CT: Appleton & Lange, 1999.

Schon LC, Myerson MS, Cuneiform-metatarsal arthrodesis for hallux valgus. In: Kitaoka HB, ed. Master techniques in orthopaedic surgery: the foot and ankle. Philadelphia: Lippincott Williams & Wilkins, 2002:99–117.

NOTES

_____
_____
_____
_____
_____
_____
_____
_____
_____
_____
_____
_____
_____

CORRECTION OF HALLUX VALGUS BY PHALANX OSTEOTOMY

CPT code   **28298 correction of hallux valgus by phalanx osteotomy**

ICD-9 code   **735.0 hallux valgus**

INDICATIONS

- as primary procedure for hallux valgus interphalangeus
- for distal metatarsal articular angle (DMAA), >12°
- as an ancillary procedure for hallux valgus

ALTERNATIVE TREATMENTS

- see CPT code 28290
- bidirectional Chevron (medial closing wedge with Chevron)

SURGICAL ANATOMY

Incision
- midline from the base of the proximal phalanx distally

APPROACHES

Surgical Techniques
- subperiosteal dissection exposing the base of the phalanx
- protect the flexor digitorum longus (FDL) and extensor hallucis longus (EHL) tendons
- a medial closing wedge osteotomy (3–4 mm)
- begin base of wedge 5–7 mm distal to metatarsal phalangeal joint
- fixation with K-wire, 1.5-mm Biofix (PLLA [polylevolactic acid]) pin, or FRS (Foot Reconstruction Set, Ace-DePuy) 2-mm break-off pin
- pin is directed from medial proximal to lateral distal

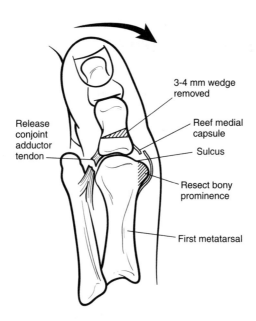

Release conjoint adductor tendon

3-4 mm wedge removed

Reef medial capsule

Sulcus

Resect bony prominence

First metatarsal

POSTOPERATIVE MANAGEMENT

- see CPT code 28290

COMPLICATIONS

- malunion/non-union
- FHL tendon rupture

SELECTED REFERENCES

Frey C. Hallux proximal phalanx osteotomy—the Akin procedure. In: Kitaoka HB, ed. Master techniques in orthopedic surgery: the foot and ankle. Philadelphia: Lippincott Williams & Wilkins, 2002:61–70.

Kelikian AS. Hallux valgus metatarsus primus varus. In: Kelikian AS, ed. Operative treatment of the foot and ankle. Stamford, CT: Appleton & Lange, 1999.

CORRECTION OF HALLUX VALGUS BY DOUBLE OSTEOTOMY

CPT code   28299 correction of hallux valgus by double osteotomy (Scarf)

ICD-9 code   735.0 hallux valgus

INDICATIONS

- moderate bunion deformity intermetatarsal angle, >15°; hallux valgus angle, >30°
- ideal for short (Morton's) first ray
- can correct abnormal distal metatarsal articular angle (DMAA)

ALTERNATIVE TREATMENTS

- Ludloff or Mau oblique shaft osteotomies
- modified Lapidus
- distal osteotomy with proximal phalanx osteotomy (Chevron/Akin)
- proximal osteotomy (dome or Chevron)

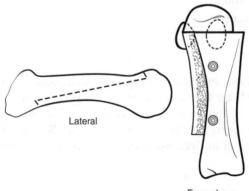

Lateral

From above

SURGICAL ANATOMY

- the osteotomy is performed proximal to the plantar neck blood supply, i.e., the medial plantar artery and the 1st intermetatarsal plantar artery
- the dorsal cutaneous nerve

Incision

- along the medial aspect of the metatarsal head in line with the shaft extending 6–7 cm proximally

APPROACHES

Surgical Techniques

- an elliptical portion of the capsule is removed along the head and neck; the adductor tenotomy is performed with a banana blade via an intra-articular approach; the fibular sesamoid is visualized by pulling the metatarsal neck proximal and the sesamoids plantar with a Ragnell to release its lateral attachments
- the septum between the abductor muscle and the medial aspect of the shaft is incised
- a Grubber guide is used
- the main osteotomy is longitudinal, from 3–4 cm in length, and oriented from dorsomedial to plantar lateral at a 15° angle
- a guide wire is placed distal, just proximal to the joint capsule 3 mm from the dorsal cortex and perpendicular to the 2nd metatarsal shaft in the frontal plane, while directing it 15° plantarward in the axial plane
- using the osteotomy guide, a proximal wire is inserted in the same orientation in the frontal and axial plane, 2–3 mm dorsal to the plantar proximal cortex
- the longitudinal cut is performed with a microsagittal long saw blade
- the proximal then distal transverse cuts are made at 60° angles: the distal cut tilted proximal and the proximal cut tilted distal
- both cuts must be oriented proximally in the frontal plane or perpendicular to the second metatarsal

- the plantar capital fragment is disengaged and translated laterally in the frontal plane up to two-thirds of its surface
- if the DMAA is high, medial tilting of the head may also be performed after resecting a 1–3 mm medial wedge of the capital fragment
- if more or less elevation of the first metatarsal is desired, the axial-plane cut is made less oblique and more transverse (elevatus) or oblique (plantar displacement)
- once the desired position has been obtained and stabilized (bone clamp) a flouroscopic check is made
- Barouk or FRS (Foot Reconstruction Set, Ace-DePuy) headless screws are used
- the distal screw is predrilled starting dorsal 1 cm from the distal cut and directed 45° obliquely distal and plantar; the drill should avoid the articular surface; the dorsal cortex is countersunk; usual screw length is 16–18 mm
- the proximal screw is placed between the proximal cut and the distal screw, starting in the midline and directed laterally and plantar; it is predrilled bicortical and then countersunk dorsally
- the resultant stepoff is shaved off medially, and the capsular closure and plication are performed medially using a running double armed 3–0 (Maxon) suture from distal to proximal in a shoelace fashion
- skin closure with 4–0 interrupted nylon
- bunion compression dressing

POSTOPERATIVE MANAGEMENT

- dressing change at 1 week and then suture removal and Velcro bunion splint at 2 weeks
- Darco OrthoWedge shoe for 3 weeks and then flat postoperative shoe for 3 weeks more
- bunion splinting is done for 4 weeks followed by toe spacer and night splinting for an additional 4 weeks
- canvas shoes at 6 weeks
- sports at 12 weeks

COMPLICATIONS

- stress fracture, <3%
- over- and undercorrection
- avascular necrosis rare
- transfer metatarsalgia rare

SELECTED REFERENCES

Barouk LS. Scarf osteotomy for hallux valgus correction. In: Myerson MS, Cracchiolo A, eds. Foot and ankle clinics. Philadelphia: WB Saunders, 2000:525–558.

NOTES

_____
_____
_____
_____
_____
_____
_____
_____
_____
_____
_____
_____

OSTEOTOMY, CALCANEUS

CPT code   28300 osteotomy; calcaneus (e.g., Dwyer or Koutsogiannis), with or
without internal fixation

ICD-9 codes   754.59 cavovarus foot (congenital)
727.68 tendon rupture of the foot and ankle nontraumatic

INDICATIONS

- deformity, either varus or valgus, of the hindfoot that is symptomatic and not responsive to orthotic devices

ALTERNATIVE TREATMENTS

- orthotic devices

SURGICAL ANATOMY

- the peroneal tendons and sural nerve lie dorsal to the skin incision

Incision

- posterior to the peroneals subtending a 45° angle to the foot; incision begins just anterior to the Achilles tendon

APPROACHES

- for a Dwyer osteotomy for cavovarus, the periosteum is elevated; 1-cm lateral closing wedge osteotomy is performed leaving the medial cortex intact; fixation is performed with a staple or axial 6.5 to 8.0-mm retrograde screw

Surgical Techniques

- the medial displacement osteotomy can be performed through the same incision for valgus deformity; the osteotomy is performed at a 45° angle to the heel using a saw; the medial cortex is also osteotomized and completed with an osteotome; the tuberosity fragment is displaced 1 cm medially; fixation is performed with an axial retrograde screw

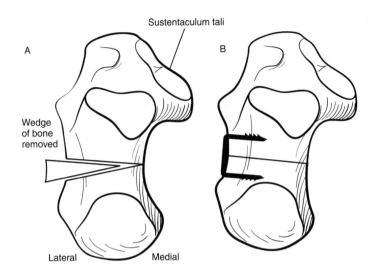

POSTOPERATIVE MANAGEMENT

- non-weight-bearing cast for 4 to 6 weeks followed by walking cast for 4 more weeks

REHABILITATION

- calf strengthening and stretching

COMPLICATIONS

- sural neuritis

SELECTED REFERENCES

Kelikian AS. Calcaneal osteotomies. In: Kelikian AS, ed. Operative treatment of the foot and ankle. Stamford, CT: Appleton & Lange, 1999:417–431.

NOTES

_____

_____

_____

_____

_____

_____

OSTEOTOMY, METATARSAL; FIRST METATARSAL

CPT code   **28306** **osteotomy with or without lengthening, shortening or angular correction, metatarsal; first metatarsal**

ICD-9 codes   **735**   **hallux valgus metatarsus primus varus (HVMTPV)**
                  735.1 **hallux varus**

INDICATIONS

- Z or Scarf osteotomy is indicated for a variety of first ray problems, the most common being HVMTPV

ALTERNATIVE TREATMENTS

- distal or proximal osteotomies

SURGICAL ANATOMY

Incision

- a linear medial incision is made from the metatarsal phalangeal joint to the base of the first metatarsal

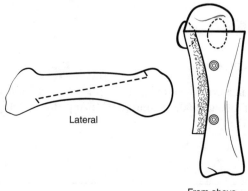

Lateral

From above

APPROACHES

Surgical Techniques

- an elliptical portion of capsule is removed over the medial aspect of the metatarsal head
- the capsule and periosteum are reflected off the shaft
- for hallux valgus, a lateral release is performed through the joint
- the osteotomy has a horizontal long diaphyseal component, which is inclined from medial to lateral 15–20 degrees directed plantarward
- once this has been completed with an oscillating saw, the distal dorsal cut is made in the metaphysis at 90° to the longitudinal osteotomy; finally the proximal plantar cut is made with a small saw blade at a 60° angle apex proximal
- using traction on the plantar capital fragment, this can be displaced laterally and angulated as well; the metatarsal shaft is then clamped
- two, 2.7-mm headless compression screws are used: one directed into the metatarsal head and the other more proximal and perpendicular to the diaphyseal long cut, which is usually 30–35 mm in length
- after redundant bone has been removed, the capsular and skin closures are performed

POSTOPERATIVE MANAGEMENT

- bulky compression dressing and splint
- a short-leg cast is applied at 2 weeks, followed by a postoperative shoe at 5 weeks for an additional 3 weeks

REHABILITATION

- active-assisted ROM, great toe

•

COMPLICATIONS

- non-union, malunion, stress fracture, and cortical/medullary invagination with over displacement

SELECTED REFERENCES

Weil LS. Scarf osteotomy for hallux valgus correction. In: Cracchiolo A, Myerson MS, eds. Foot and ankle clinics: the hallux. Philadelphia: WB Saunders, 2000:559–580.

NOTES

_____
_____
_____
_____
_____
_____
_____
_____
_____
_____
_____

OSTEOTOMY, METATARSAL; OTHER THAN THE FIRST

CPT code   **28308 osteotomy with or without lengthening, shortening or angular correction, metatarsal; other than the first, each (e.g., Weil type)**

ICD-9 code   **726.70 metatarsalgia**

INDICATIONS

- central or isolated metatarsalgia
- transfer lesion
- claw or varus toe deformity in conjunction with a tendon transfer (CPT code 27690)

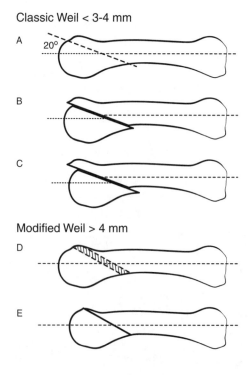

Classic Weil < 3-4 mm

A   20°

B

C

Modified Weil > 4 mm

D

E

ALTERNATIVE TREATMENTS

- orthotic devices
- metatarsal pads
- metatarsal shoe bars
- Budin pads
- DuVries condylectomy (CPT code 28288)

SURGICAL ANATOMY

Incision
- dorsal interdigital space, linear, 3–4 cm

APPROACHES

Surgical Techniques
- after retracting the extensor mechanism by developing the interval between the short and long toe extensor tendon, the head and neck of the metatarsal are exposed
- the capsule is divided transversely
- small Hohmann retractors are placed around the metatarsal neck
- a McGlamry skid is placed plantar to retract the toe plantar
- a long microsagittal saw blade is used
- an oblique (20° to the shaft) osteotomy is begun distally, beginning on the dorsal articular surface
- the blade is advanced proximally, parallel to the plantar surface of the foot
- usual shortening is 3–4 mm
- if more shortening is needed, then a modification is done resecting a dorsal distal wedge from the shaft
- fixation is with a 1.6-mm threaded pin, or a 2-mm (Foot Reconstruction Set, Ace-DePuy) snap off screw

POSTOPERATIVE MANAGEMENT

- Darco OrthoWedge shoe for 3 weeks
- active and passive toe-flexion exercises (10 repetitions, three times per day)

COMPLICATIONS

- loss of plantar flexion
- transfer lesions

SELECTED REFERENCES

Davies MS, Saxby TS. Metatarsal neck osteotomy with rigid fixation for the treatment of lesser toe metatarsal phalangeal pathology. Foot Ankle Int 1999;20:630–635.

NOTES

_____
_____
_____
_____
_____
_____
_____
_____
_____
_____
_____

SESAMOIDECTOMY, FIRST TOE (SEPARATE PROCEDURE)

CPT code   28315 sesamoidectomy, first toe (separate procedure)

ICD-9 code   733.99 sesamoiditis

INDICATIONS

- painful non-union of tibial or fibular sesamoid
- arthritis of sesamoid complex
- avascular necrosis of sesamoid

ALTERNATIVE TREATMENTS

- orthotic devices
- dancer's pads
- open reduction—internal fixation (ORIF) for fracture and bone graft for non-union

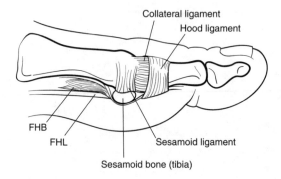

Collateral ligament
Hood ligament
FHB
FHL
Sesamoid ligament
Sesamoid bone (tibia)

SURGICAL ANATOMY

Incision
- for fibular sesamoid, a dorsal approach between the first and second interdigital spaces
- alternatively, plantar on the lateral side of the fibular sesamoid
- straight medial incision centered over the medial eminence for the tibial sesamoid

APPROACHES

Surgical Techniques
- if the intermetatarsal angle is high, then the dorsal approach allows for access
- laminar spreader facilitates exposure
- the fibular sesamoid lies at the level of the metatarsal neck
- an Allis, Kocher, or loose body clamp is placed axially on the sesamoid
- a no. 67 Beaver blade is used to peel off the ligamentous flexor brevis attachments
- care is taken to avoid injury to the flexor hallucis longus (FHL) tendon
- for the plantar approach, a small curvilinear incision is made
- the digital neurovascular bundle and FHL tendon are avoided
- for the tibial sesamoid, the abductor tendon and capsule are incised via medial approach
- the sesamoid is identified plantar and excised as described previously
- after excision, the brevis tendon ends are brought together with a 2–0 nonabsorbable suture

POSTOPERATIVE MANAGEMENT

- stiff-soled shoe, 4 weeks
- avoid dorsiflexion exercises
- tibial excision—use bunion-type splinting to avoid hallux valgus
- for fibular excision, splint the toe in valgus to avoid varus
- splint for 4 weeks

COMPLICATIONS

- hallux valgus for tibial excision (perform osteotomy if preexisting hallux valgus)
- hallux varus for fibular excision
- cock-up deformity—avoid excising both sesamoids
- digital neuroma

SELECTED REFERENCES

Kelikian H. The sesamoids. In: Kelikian H. Hallux valgus and allied deformities of the forefoot including metatarsalgia. Philadelphia: WB Saunders, 1965.

NOTES

_____
_____
_____
_____
_____
_____
_____
_____
_____
_____
_____

REPAIR, NON-UNION OR MALUNION, TARSAL BONES

CPT code   28320 repair, non-union or malunion; tarsal bones

ICD-9 code   733.82 non-union fracture

INDICATIONS

- non-union or malunion of talar neck fractures without subtalar arthritis

ALTERNATIVE TREATMENTS

- subtalar or triple arthrodesis

SURGICAL ANATOMY

- with talar neck non-union and malunion, the capital fragment is usually in varus and extension; this requires the tricortical bone graft to be placed dorsal and medial

Incision

- anteromedial over the neck of the talus in the interval between the anterior tibial (AT) and posterior tibial (PT) tendons.
- if need for joint reduction, a separate sinus tarsi approach is used (CPT code 28116)

APPROACHES

Surgical Techniques

- a 6.5 to 8.0-mm cancellous screw is placed from posterolateral to anteromedial antegrade into the talar head

POSTOPERATIVE MANAGEMENT

- non-weight-bearing splint for 2 weeks
- non-weight-bearing cast for 4 more weeks followed by exercises

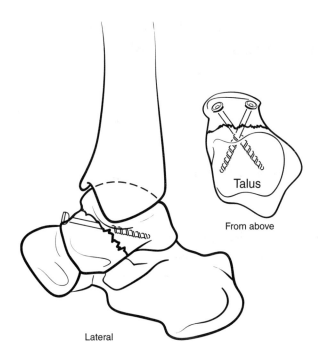

Talus

From above

Lateral

REHABILITATION

- a weight-bearing brace is allowed when there is radiographic union (10–16 weeks)

COMPLICATIONS

- non-union and subtalar arthritis

SELECTED REFERENCES

Kelikian AS. Talus fractures. In: Kelikian AS, ed. Operative treatment of the foot and ankle. Stamford, CT: Appleton & Lange, 1999:495–515.

NOTES

_____
_____
_____
_____
_____

PERCUTANEOUS SKELETAL FIXATION OF CALCANEAL FRACTURE, WITH MANIPULATION

CPT code   28406 percutaneous skeletal fixation of calcaneal fracture, with manipulation

ICD-9 code   282.80 fracture tarsal foot, calcaneus

INDICATIONS

- displaced intra-articular fractures, calcaneus
- displaced extra-articular fractures, calcaneus—beak type
- not amenable to open fixation—internal fixation (ORIF) (type IV)

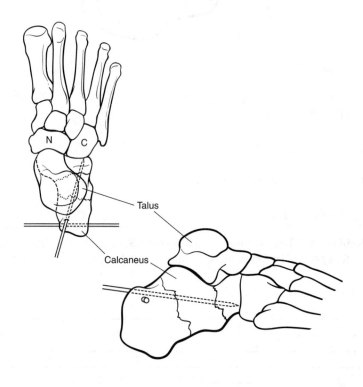

ALTERNATIVE TREATMENTS

- nonoperative: ROM and non-weight-bearing
- small pin fixator with circular frame
- ORIF

SURGICAL ANATOMY

Incision
- percutaneous

APPROACHES

Surgical Techniques
- lateral decubitus or prone (bilateral)
- large Steinmann pin through tuberosity
- attach to Charnley traction bow
- manual or 20-lb sterile traction off distal table with pulley
- axial traction pin (Essex-Lopresti)
- percutaneous large pin lateral to elevate joint compression fracture
- axial pins may be changed out for large (6.5 to 8-mm) cannulated screws
- superior lateral joint fragment can be stabilized with 4-mm cannulated cancellous screws
- beak fractures can be stabilized with large cancellous screws and washer
- large Schanz screw in tuberosity instead of transverse for tongue-type fractures

POSTOPERATIVE MANAGEMENT

- bulky compression dressing and posterior splint for 2 weeks
- for beak fractures, 6 weeks equinus non-weight-bearing cast
- at 10 weeks, weight bearing if x-rays show consolidation

COMPLICATIONS

- fat pad atrophy
- peroneal impingement
- subtalar arthritis
- loss of reduction

SELECTED REFERENCES

Forgon M. Closed reduction and percutaneous osteosynthesis in 265 calcaneus fractures. In: Tscherne T, Schatzker J. Major fractures of the pilon, talus, and calcaneus. New York: Springer, 1993:207–213.

Hansen ST. Functional reconstruction of the foot and ankle. Philadelphia: Lippincott Williams & Wilkins, 2000:80–84.

NOTES

_____

_____

_____

_____

_____

_____

_____

_____

_____

_____

_____

_____

_____

OPEN TREATMENT OF CALCANEAL FRACTURE

CPT code   28415 open treatment of calcaneal fracture, with or without internal
                        or external fixation, each

ICD-9 code   825.0 fracture calcaneus (closed)

INDICATIONS

- displaced intra-articular fractures (Sander's grade II–III), with displacement of more than 2 mm, articular malalignment of >10°, or tuberosity translation >1 cm. Displaced beak (extra-articular posterior tuberosity) fractures as well

ALTERNATIVE TREATMENTS

- nonoperative with early ROM
- delayed fusion with open reduction—internal fixation ORIF for type IV
- Ilizarov for type IV

SURGICAL ANATOMY

- the extensile L flap (Dwyer) is based upon the peroneal arterioles and venules
- surgery should be delayed 7–21 days until there is a lateral "wrinkle sign"

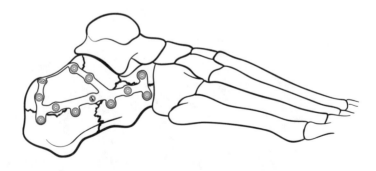

Incision

- the vertical limb is 1 cm anterior to the Achilles and extends distally to where it forms a juncture with the horizontal limb, which is about 2 cm above the plantar skin

APPROACHES

- the sural nerve is protected at each end of the incision
- the patient is placed in a decubitus position for unilateral cases, and prone position for bilateral cases

SURGICAL TECHNIQUES

- the flap is elevated subperiosteally using a no-touch technique
- 1.6-mm K-wires are placed in the cuboid, talus, and fibula to retract the flap
- a 3.2-mm K-wire is placed in the corner of the flap from lateral to medial, and attached to a Charnley clamp for distal traction on the tuberosity to disengage it from the superolateral (joint fragment) and the constant sustentacular piece
- the superolateral fragment is reduced and transfixed with a K-wire from the 4-mm cannulated screw set
- after the joint has been fixed with one to two cancellous screws, a lateral calcaneal buttress plate is applied and fixed to span the anterior and posterior columns of the calcaneus—make sure that the hindfoot (tuberosity) is aligned and held with a temporary 2-mm K-wire
- final lateral, axial, and Broden's views are taken and checked

POSTOPERATIVE MANAGEMENT

- bulky compression dressing
- sutures removed at 3 weeks
- ROM is begun to include inversion/eversion, pronation/supination, and ankle flexion/extension

REHABILITATION

- non-weight-bearing cast for 8–10 weeks

COMPLICATIONS

- marginal skin necrosis
- implant irritation, arthrosis, and sural neuritis

SELECTED REFERENCES

Kelikian AS, Jimenez ML. Fractures of the calcaneus. In: Kelikian AS, ed. Operative treatment of the foot and ankle. Stamford, CT: Appleton & Lange, 1999:389–416.

NOTES

OPEN TREATMENT OF METATARSAL FRACTURE

CPT code   **28485** open treatment of metatarsal fracture, with or without internal fixation, each

ICD-9 code   **825.25** metatarsus of one foot, closed

INDICATIONS

- displaced first metatarsal
- lesser metatarsals with sagittal plane angulation
- fifth metatarsal: Jones fracture (2 cm proximal to the base), stress fracture of the proximal metaphyseal—diaphyseal junction, delayed unions

ALTERNATIVE TREATMENTS

- nonoperative non-weight-bearing cast for 6–8 weeks, then short-leg weight-bearing cast for an additional 6–8 weeks for fifth metatarsal

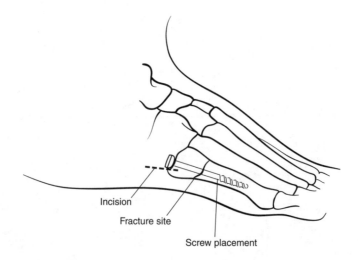

Incision

Fracture site

Screw placement

SURGICAL ANATOMY

Incision
- linear, medial to long toe extensor
- for fifth metatarsal, percutaneous at base of fifth metatarsal and extend proximal 2–3 cm

APPROACHES

Surgical Techniques
- patient is in a semi-decubitus position
- for fifth metatarsal, a guide wire is inserted under fluoroscopic control high and inside relative to the tuberosity
- check the wire position on anterior-posterior, lateral, internal, and oblique views
- use appropriate-sized drill, and countersink and tap the bone if required
- screw size can range from 4.5 to 6.5 mm depending on the canal size
- the length is dependent on the fracture location and is usually between 50 and 65 mm
- for diaphyseal metatarsal fractures, use small or mini-fragment plates (locking in osteoporotic bone)
- for open fractures, consider mini external fixator
- for neck fractures, percutaneous K-wire antegrade then retrograde
- for delayed or non-union, consider cancellous bone graft

POSTOPERATIVE MANAGEMENT

- with intramedullary screws, non-weight-bearing for 2 weeks, then CAM walker for 4 weeks
- return to sports when consolidation—usually no sooner than 10–12 weeks
- for plates, non-weight-bearing 4–6 weeks, then full weight bearing with cast or CAM walker for 4 weeks more
- for K-wires, as described previously but remove pin by 6 weeks

COMPLICATIONS

- non-union
- hardware failure

SELECTED REFERENCES

Kodros SA. In: Stern SH, ed. Key techniques in orthopedic surgery. New
    York: Thieme Medical Publishers, 2001:260–262.
Trevino SG, Williams RL, Stiff TE. Lisfranc and proximal fifth metatarsal
    injuries. In: Kelikian AS, ed. Operative treatment of the foot and ankle.
    Stamford, CT: Appleton & Lange, 1999:479–491.

NOTES

_____
_____
_____
_____
_____
_____
_____
_____
_____
_____
_____

ARTHRODESIS, PANTALAR

CPT code   28705 Arthrodesis, pantalar

ICD-9 codes   716.97 arthritis, osteoarthritis foot & ankle
                    714   rheumatoid arthritis, RA
                    713.57 Charcot, foot and ankle

INDICATIONS

- arthritis or deformity involving the tibiotalocalcaneal (TTC) joints as well as the Chopart (talonavicular and calcaneocuboid) joints

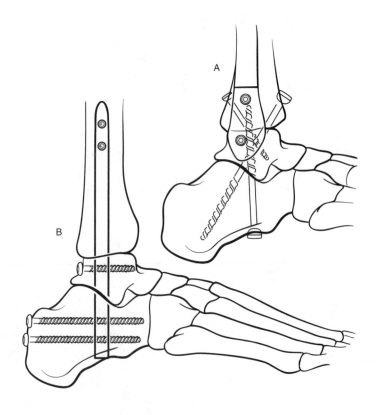

ALTERNATIVE TREATMENTS

- ankle–foot orthosis (AFO)
- calcaneal retaining orthotic walker (CROW)
- below-the-knee amputation
- various fixation methods available for fusion: retrograde intramedullary locked nails, blade plates (humeral), external fixator (circular), locking plates, and multiple screws

SURGICAL ANATOMY

Incision
- posterolateral 15-cm length for TTC joint
- lateral for the TTC joint (transfibular)
- distal sinus tarsi for the calcaneocuboid joint
- medial linear between the anterior tibial and posterior tibial tendons

APPROACHES

Surgical Techniques
- prone when using the posterolateral
- supine when using lateral
- when prone, develop the plane between the flexor hallucis longus (FHL) and peroneal tendons
- when supine, the distal 5 cm of fibula is resected, then morcellized for bone graft
- iliac or allograft chips may be mixed with autogenous growth factor (AGF) when prone
- the Chopart joints are exposed if they need to be included in the fusion, then decorticated
- the TTC joints are prepared using ring curettes and large 6-mm burr
- laminar spreader for visualization
- correct any deformity prior to fixation
- using the retrograde nail (Versa nail—Ace-DePuy or Biomet), a guide pin is inserted
- at the anterior portion of the heel pad in line with the second and third web spaces in the sagittal plane into the tibia

- fluoroscopic verification is done in the anteroposterior, lateral, and axial planes
- a transverse, 2-cm incision is made and bluntly developed
- trocar manual reamer is introduced retrograde from the heel into the tibia
- a guide pin is placed; then sequential flexible reamers beginning at 9 mm and ending 0.5 mm larger than the final nail diameter
- reaming depth should be 2-cm greater than the final nail length (to compensate for heel-pad thickness)
- the external jig attaches to the appropriate-sized nail (10 or 12 mm × 150–300 mm)
- the screws may be aligned medial/lateral or posterior/anterior
- the posterior/anterior construct allows for better purchase in the calcaneus and talus, as well as the versatility to include the Chopart joints if needed; the jig is rotated from posterior to medial
- two ½-inch pins are then placed in the proximal tibia medially to facilitate compression through the jig
- the proximal screws are predrilled and placed from medial to lateral into the tibia
- fluoroscopic check is made; then the jig is removed—onlay bone graft is performed and then routine closure

POSTOPERATIVE MANAGEMENT

- posterior plaster coaptation splint for 2 weeks
- sutures removed then short-leg cast, non-weight-bearing
- in non-neuropathic patients, weight-bearing cast from weeks 4 to 8 and then CAM walker for 4 weeks
- in neuropathic patients, total-contact cast, non-weight-bearing (change every 2 weeks), until week 8; then weight-bearing cast for 8 more weeks
- long-term shoe prescription for rocker bottom sole

COMPLICATIONS

- non-union; implant bursitis; proximal tibial stress fracture
- infection
- eccentric entry site in heel with cutting out
- neuropraxia of posterior tibial nerve from plantar portal site

SELECTED REFERENCES

Kelikian AS. Ankle arthrodesis. In: Kelikian AS, ed. Operative treatment of the foot and ankle. Stamford, CT: Appleton & Lange, 1999.

NOTES

_____

_____

_____

_____

_____

_____

_____

_____

_____

_____

_____

_____

_____

ARTHRODESIS, TRIPLE

CPT code   28715 arthrodesis, triple

ICD-9 codes   716.97 arthritis, osteoarthritis, foot and ankle
                     714   rheumatoid arthritis, RA
                     726.72 posterior tibial dysfunction, stage III–IV

INDICATIONS

- arthritis involving the subtalar and Chopart joints
- arthritis with deformity
- paralytic (poliomyelitis)

ALTERNATIVE TREATMENTS

- orthotic devices
- Arizona brace

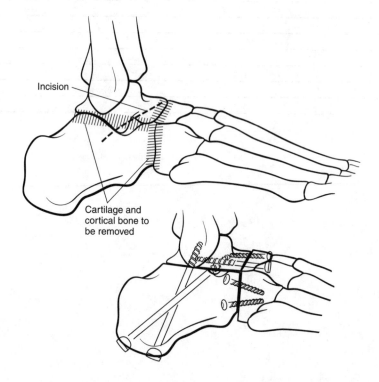

SURGICAL ANATOMY

- see CPT code 28725

Incision
- a separate linear incision is made in the interval between the anterior and posterior tibial tendons, beginning 2 cm distal to the medial malleolus

APPROACHES

- an Ollier sinus tarsi lateral approach is made extending distal past the anterior process, 4 cm
- see CPT code 28725

Surgical Techniques
- after decorticating the subtalar joint expose the calcaneocuboid joint by elevating the extensor digitorum brevis
- with an oscillating saw, remove 2–3 mm on each side of the joint
- for the talonavicular joint, protect the tibial tendons
- use curved osteotomes or gouges to retain the convex shape of the talar head
- for the navicular, decorticate with a curette and then a 6-mm burr to keep the concave surface
- correct any deformity of the talar inclination or declination prior to temporary stabilization with guide pins
- for fixation, use a 7.3 or 8-mm retrograde cancellous screw for the subtalar joint
- use a retrograde 6.5-mm screw for the talonavicular joint
- for the calcaneocuboid joint, use either two cross 5-mm cancellous screws, Uniclip staples (Wright Medical), or a combination of the two
- the foot should be plantigrade, neutral-to-slight pronation, and the heel in 5° of valgus
- cancellous bone graft is optional as indicated
- if the ankle is in any residual equinus after deformity correction perform a tendo Achilles lengthening (TAL) (CPT 27606)

POSTOPERATIVE MANAGEMENT

- posterior mold with coaptation splint and bulky compression dressing
- sutures removed at 2–3 weeks
- non-weight-bearing short-leg cast for another 2–3 weeks, followed by walking cast for 4–5 weeks more

COMPLICATIONS

- non-union/malunion
- incisional neuroma
- late ipsilateral ankle arthritis

SELECTED REFERENCES

Quill G. Subtalar reconstruction. In: Kelikian AS, ed. Operative treatment of the foot and ankle. Stamford, CT: Appleton & Lange, 1999:433–454.

NOTES

_____
_____
_____
_____
_____
_____
_____
_____
_____
_____

ARTHRODESIS, SUBTALAR

CPT code   **28725 subtalar arthrodesis**

ICD-9 code   **716.97 arthritis, foot and ankle (subtalar)**

INDICATIONS

- subtalar joint arthritis—degenerative, inflammatory, posttraumatic
- coalition, middle facet
- posterior tibial dysfunction

ALTERNATIVE TREATMENTS

- NSAIDs, corticosteroid injections
- orthotic devices (UCBL)

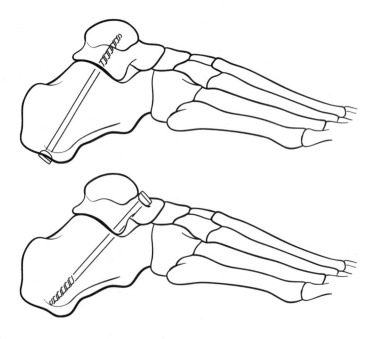

SURGICAL ANATOMY

Incision
- Ollier over the sinus tarsi in Langer's skin line
- posterolateral

APPROACHES

Surgical Techniques
- avoid the sural nerve posterior to the peroneal tendons as well as the intermediate branch of the superficial peroneal nerve; retract the peroneals with a Z retractor
- debride the sinus tarsi
- place a laminar spreader in the sinus and distract the talus and calcaneus
- remove the remaining cartilage on the apposing talocalcaneal surfaces with a ring curette; then burr (6 mm) to bleeding bone on all three facets
- place a guide pin retrograde in the mid-axial line (second to third webspace) in the heel, then an antegrade pin in the talar neck
- place the heel in 5° of exorotation (valgus) and engage the pins across the joint
- prior to drilling, check axial and lateral views with the fluoroscope
- drill the outer cortices; countersink the heel
- place allograft or autograft between the joint surfaces in a moldable fashion
- use either 6.5-, 7.3-, or 8-mm cancellous screws
- close the wound in interrupted layers
- for the posterolateral approach, position the patient in the decubitus position on a bean bag with the affected side up
- make an 8-cm incision, centered over the subtalar joint, and begin just anterior to the Achilles
- identify the flexor hallucis longus (FHL) tendon crossing from lateral to medial beginning proximally
- retract the FHL medially and the peroneals laterally
- debride the joint in the manner previously described using a laminar spreader posterior as well

- use two retrograde, fully threaded cancellous 6.5-mm screws for bone block arthrodesis
- use the cross screws with moldable graft for other cases

POSTOPERATIVE MANAGEMENT

- non-weight-bearing splint, 2 weeks
- sutures removed and cast changed at 2 weeks
- weight-bearing cast at 4 weeks
- CAM walker at 8 weeks
- for bone block arthrodesis, non-weight-bearing 10 weeks and then CAM walker

COMPLICATIONS

- non-union, 10%
- incisional neuroma

SELECTED REFERENCES

Quill G. Subtalar reconstruction. In: Kelikian AS, ed. Operative treatment of the foot and ankle. Stamford, CT: Appleton & Lange, 1999:433–454.

NOTES

_____
_____
_____
_____
_____
_____
_____
_____
_____
_____

ARTHRODESIS, MIDTARSAL OR TARSOMETATARSAL, MULTIPLE OR TRANSVERSE

CPT code   **28730 arthrodesis; midtarsal or tarsometatarsal, multiple or transverse**

ICD-9 code   **716.97 arthritis of the foot**

INDICATIONS

- pain not responsive to medical and pedorthotic management

ALTERNATIVE TREATMENTS

- orthotic devices
- rocker bottom shoes with extended steel shank
- NSAIDs

SURGICAL ANATOMY

- the relationship between the neurovascular bundle and the extensor hallucis longus (EHL), extensor hallucis brevis (EHB), and extensor digitorum communis (EDC) tendons

Incision

- the first and second tarsometatarsal joints are approached in the interval between the EHL and EHB tendons
- the second and third tarsometatarsal joints are approached between the EDC and EHB
- the talonavicular joint is exposed between the anterior tibial and posterior tibial tendons, whereas the calcaneocuboid (CC) joint is exposed at the level of the anterior calcaneal process just above the peroneal tendons

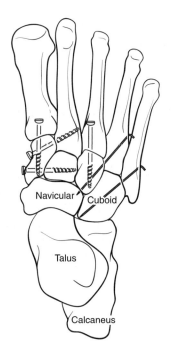

APPROACHES

Surgical Techniques

- decortication is performed with a small sagittal saw, rasp, and rongeur for the talometatarsal and CC joints
- the convex–concave relationship of the talonavicular joint is retained by using a gouge and burr
- fixation for the talometatarsal joint is via retrograde 4-mm cancellous screws
- the CC joint is stabilized with staples or cross 5-mm screws, whereas the talonavicular joint is fixed with an axial 6.5-mm screw and/or staples

POSTOPERATIVE MANAGEMENT

- non-weight-bearing cast, 4 weeks
- full weight-bearing cast, 4 weeks

REHABILITATION

- strengthening exercises

COMPLICATIONS

- non-union, 10% (2–3 times more in smokers)

SELECTED REFERENCES

Mann RA. Treatment of primary arthrosis of the midtarsal and
   tarsometatarsal joints. In: Myerson MS, ed. Foot and ankle clinics:
   arthrodesis procedures. Philadelphia: WB Saunders, 1996:85–92.
Schon LC, Bell W. Fusions of the transverse tarsal and midtarsal joints. In:
   Myerson MS, ed. Foot and ankle clinics: arthrodesis procedure.
   Philadelphia: WB Saunders, 1996:93–108.

NOTES

_____

_____

_____

_____

_____

_____

_____

_____

_____

_____

_____

ARTHRODESIS, MIDTARSAL OR TARSOMETATARSAL, MULTIPLE TRANSVERSE WITH OSTEOTOMY

CPT code   28735 arthrodesis; midtarsal or tarsometatarsal, multiple transverse
                          with osteotomy (e.g., flatfoot correction)

ICD-9 codes   713.5 Charcot joint disease
                   734   pes planus

INDICATIONS

- Charcot arthropathy with midfoot collapse "at risk" with rocker bottom deformity
- posttraumatic arthritis
- painful flatfoot, not responsive to conservative measures

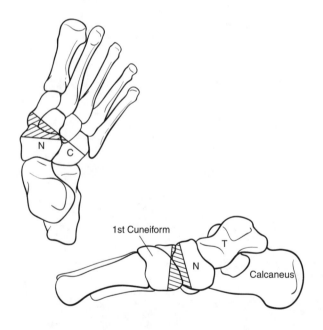

ALTERNATIVE TREATMENTS

- extra-depth shoes with rocker bottom soles
- orthotic devices (trilayer with plastizoate for patients with neuropathy)
- exostectomy

SURGICAL ANATOMY

Incision
- extensile extended medial approach (Henry)
- lateral over the calcaneocuboid (CC) joint

APPROACHES

Surgical Techniques
- all dissection is kept subperiosteal
- maintain the peroneal and anterior tibial tendons
- for rocker bottom, a plantar-based wedge-resection fusion is done at the affected joint, i.e., tarsometatarsal, naviculo cuneiform, or talonavicular
- in the frontal plane, a medial wedge is removed for valgus, and a lateral-based wedge for varus deformity
- fixation can be with large fragment axial screws
- if possible, plantar pre-bent locking plates
- tendo Achilles lengthening (TAL) if needed

POSTOPERATIVE MANAGEMENT

- total-contact cast (TCC) for neuropathic cases
- change every 2 weeks
- non-weight-bearing for 8 weeks then full weight-bearing TCC for and additional 8 weeks

COMPLICATIONS

- non-union
- malunion
- hardware failure

- infection
- recurrent ulceration
- delayed wound healing

SELECTED REFERENCES

Sangeorzan BJ, Hansen ST. Cuneiform-metatarsal (Lisfranc) arthrodesis. In: Kitaoka HB, ed. Master techniques in orthopaedic surgery: the foot and ankle. Philadelphia: Lippincott Williams & Wilkins, 2002:237–252.
Schon LC, Bell W. Fusions of the transverse tarsal and midtarsal joints. In: Myerson MS, ed. Foot and ankle clinics. Philadelphia: WB Saunders, 1996:93–108.

NOTES

ARTHRODESIS, GREAT TOE; METATARSAL PHALANGEAL JOINT

CPT code   28750 arthrodesis, great toe; metatarsal phalangeal joint

ICD-9 code   735.2 hallux rigidus, acquired

INDICATIONS

- stage II–III hallux rigidus
- failed bunion surgery
- neuromuscular bunions
- inflammatory arthritis

ALTERNATIVE TREATMENTS

- stiff-soled shoes
- Morton's extension carbon fiber orthotic devices
- osteotomies
- implant arthroplasty
- Keller resection arthroplasty

SURGICAL ANATOMY

Incision

- dorsal just medial to the extensor hallucis longus (EHL) tendon centered over the metatarsal phalangeal joint (CPT code 28289)
- medial linear (CPT code 28290)

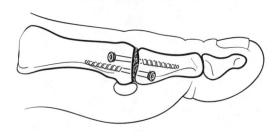

APPROACHES

Surgical Techniques

- expose the metatarsal phalangeal joint
- retract the EHL tendon lateral
- the remaining articular cartilage is removed with a rongeur
- the Acumed reamer system is used
- a 1.6-mm K-wire is placed retrograde up the metatarsal shaft
- a large concave reamer is used to remove the sclerotic bone
- next the K-wire is placed antegrade down the proximal phalanx axis
- the small convex reamer deepens the surface and the large one widens it
- a 4-mm burr can be used for fine tuning
- the hallux is positioned in 10° of valgus, 0° rotation, and 10–15° of dorsiflexion relative to the floor (females in 15°)
- two cross K-wires are inserted from the cannulated set (medial to lateral, one antegrade and one retrograde)
- after fluoroscopic check, the 2.9-mm cannulated drill is used
- with cortical screws, the near cortex is overdrilled with a 3.5-mm bit or short cancellous 4-mm screws are used
- solid screws are preferred
- bone reamings are placed dorsally prior to closure

POSTOPERATIVE MANAGEMENT

- Darco OrthoWedge shoe for 4 weeks—flat-soled wooden shoe for 4 weeks
- sports at 12 weeks

COMPLICATIONS

- non-union, 10%
- malunion

SELECTED REFERENCES

Kelikian AS. Hallux valgus metatarsus primus varus. In: Kelikian AS, ed. Operative treatment of the foot and ankle. Stamford, CT: Appleton & Lange, 1999.

ARTHRODESIS, GREAT TOE; INTERPHALANGEAL JOINT

CPT code   28755 arthrodesis, great toe; interphalangeal joint

ICD-9 code   715.17 arthritis, foot and ankle

INDICATIONS

- arthritis of the interphalangeal joint of the great toe, either posttraumatic or inflammatory
- fusion in conjunction with extensor hallucis longus (EHL) transfer for hallux varus corrective surgery
- mallet toe deformity of great toe

ALTERNATIVE TREATMENTS

- see CPT code 28750 (Chapter 54)

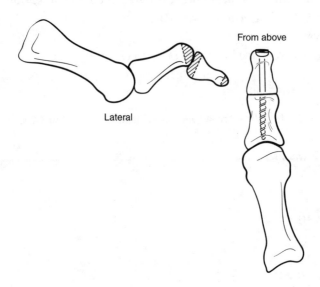

From above

Lateral

SURGICAL ANATOMY

Incision
- transverse at interphalangeal joint and proximal medial longitudinal as well as distal lateral limb if needed

APPROACHES

Surgical Techniques
- transection of EHL tendon
- remove 2 mm on each side of joint with an oscillating saw
- fixation with a 4.5-mm, 5.0-mm, or $^4/_5$-mm (Acumed) lag screw in a retrograde fashion
- for hallux varus, the EHL tendon is re-routed plantar under the transverse intermetatarsal (IM) ligament via a drill hole on the lateral base of the proximal phalanx
- another option is to detach the tendon proximally and then re-route it from distal to proximal and lateral to medial through the first metatarsal neck via an oblique drill hole after going plantar to the transverse IM ligament

POSTOPERATIVE MANAGEMENT

- stiff-soled postoperative shoe for 4 weeks

COMPLICATIONS

- non-union

SELECTED REFERENCES

Hansen ST. Functional reconstruction of the foot and ankle. Philadelphia: Lippincott Willliams & Wilkins, 2000.

TRANSMETATARSAL AMPUTATION

CPT code   28805 transmetatarsal amputation

ICD-9 codes   443.9 peripheral vascular disease
                    730.1 osteomyelitis—chronic

INDICATIONS

- intact plantar skin in the face of gangrene or osteomyelitis of the toes or distal metatarsals
- posttraumatic open degloving injuries
- contraindicated in non-ambulators
- recurrent neuropathic forefoot ulcers

ALTERNATIVE TREATMENTS

- Syme's or below-the-knee amputation
- Hoffmann head resections

SURGICAL ANATOMY

Incision
- fish mouth dorsal and plantar flaps with the plantar one being longer

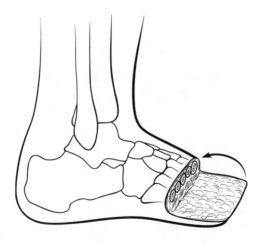

APPROACHES

Surgical Techniques
- dorsal flap is developed full-thickness to the metatarsals
- the anterior tibial artery and vein are ligated
- all tendons are cut under tension
- the plantar flap, which is longer, is developed subperiosteally with an elevator
- the flexor tendons are cut under tension
- the metatarsals are cut with an oscillating saw beveled from dorsal to plantar
- the normal declination angle of the metatarsals from 1–5 is preserved, i.e., the medial rays are just longer than the adjacent lateral ones
- the flaps are closed, interrupted under minimal tension

POSTOPERATIVE MANAGEMENT

- bulky compression dressing with a plaster mold
- sutures remain for 4 weeks
- postoperative wooden plastizoate-lined shoe or CAM walker from 3–6 weeks
- extra-depth shoe with end filler insole

COMPLICATIONS

- neuroma
- failed wound healing

SELECTED REFERENCES

Brodsky JW. Transmetatarsal amputation. In: Kitaoka HB, ed. Master techniques in orthopaedic surgery: the foot and ankle. New York: Lippincott Williams &Wilkins, 2002:221–236.

APPLICATION OF RIGID TOTAL-CONTACT LEG CAST

CPT code   29445 application of rigid total-contact leg cast

ICD-9 codes   094.0   Charcot's arthropathy (also 713.5)
                  707.15 diabetic ulcer of the foot

INDICATIONS

- ambulatory treatment of plantar ulcers of neuropathic feet; contraindicated in face of infection or severe ischemia
- neuropathic joints and fractures, as well as postoperative immobilization

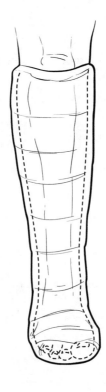

ALTERNATIVE TREATMENTS

- local wound care with orthotic devices, CROW brace, or Aircast walking boot

SURGICAL ANATOMY

- peripheral neuropathy leads to diminished sensation, which allows excessive and prolonged pressure that leads to skin breakdown— deformity can also play a role

Incision

- ulcer is debrided locally as is the callus; a sterile, nonadhesive dressing is applied

APPROACHES

Surgical Techniques

- after applying a stockinette, which is cut anteriorly about the ankle, a single layer of 50% overlapping 4-inch Webril cast padding is applied from the tibial tubercle to the tips of the toes
- a 1 × 4-cm piece of ¼-inch felt is placed from the tubercle to the ankle; additional pieces are placed over the malleoli as well as around the toes
- a single layer of plaster is applied followed by fiberglass tape—the foot and ankle as well as the arch are molded

POSTOPERATIVE MANAGEMENT

- cast shoe for ambulation; the first cast is changed at 1 week, and then every 2 weeks
- when the ulcer is healed (6–16 weeks) proper pedorthic footwear and inserts are applied for fractures and postoperative use; radiographic consolidation should be a guide; this is usually greater than two times in the sensate patient

COMPLICATIONS

- recurrent ulceration can be 20–30%

SELECTED REFERENCES

Dhawan S, Conti SF. Use of total contact casting in the diabetic foot. In: Brodsky JW, Myerson MS. Foot and ankle clinics: the diabetic foot. Philadelphia: WB Saunders, 1997:1115–1134.

NOTES

_____

_____

_____

_____

_____

_____

_____

_____

_____

_____

_____

ARTHROSCOPY, ANKLE, SURGICAL; EXCISION OF OSTEOCHONDRAL DEFECT

CPT code   **29891 arthroscopy, ankle, surgical; excision of osteochondral defect of talus and/or tibia, including drilling of the defect**

ICD-9 code   **732.5 osteochondral lesion of the talus**

INDICATIONS

- failed conservative treatment

ALTERNATIVE TREATMENTS

- for Brendt and Harty stage I–II lesions (and stage III lesions in children), weight-bearing cast is recommended (6–10 weeks); arthroscopy is then advocated if symptomatic and for all stage III–IV lesions evident on computed tomography (CT)/magnetic resonance imaging (MRI)
- acute lesions with an osseous fragment should be reattached with absorbable pins, screws, or K-wires
- chronic lesions are debrided and treated with microfracture technique via drilling to a 10-mm depth with a 1.6-mm K-wire
- failed surgical cases or large lesions can be treated with osteoarticular transplants (OATs)

SURGICAL ANATOMY

- lateral lesions are usually anterior, whereas medial ones are more posterior

Incision
- anteromedial, anterolateral, and posterolateral portals (CPT code 29898)

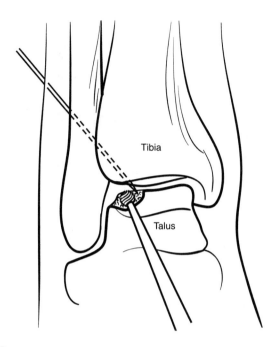

APPROACHES

- arthroscopic in most cases; seldom transmalleolar osteotomy is indicated or plafondplasty

Surgical Techniques

- small instruments, 2.7-mm scope, 2.9-mm shaver, pressure inflow, noninvasive distractor, and vector guide are all useful armamentarium

POSTOPERATIVE MANAGEMENT

- sutures and splint for 7–10 days

REHABILITATION

- non-weight-bearing for 4 weeks (7 weeks for OATs)

COMPLICATIONS

- neuropraxia, 10%

SELECTED REFERENCES

Assenmacher JA, Kelikian AS, Gottlob C, Kodros S. Arthroscopically assisted autologous osteochondral transplantation for osteochondral lesions of the talar dome: an MRI and clinical follow-up study. Foot Ankle Int 2001;22:544–551.

Ferkel RD, Cheng JC. Ankle and subtalar arthroscopy. In: Kelikian AS, ed. Operative treatment of the foot and ankle. Stamford, CT: Appleton & Lange, 1999:321–350.

Hangody L. Mosaicplasty for the treatment of osteochondritis dissecans of the talus: two to seven year results in 36 patients. Foot Ankle Int 2001;22:552–558.

NOTES

ARTHROSCOPY, ANKLE, SURGICAL; WITH EXTENSIVE DEBRIDEMENT

CPT code   **29898 arthroscopy, ankle, (tibiotalar and fibulotalar joints), surgical; with debridement extensive**

ICD-9 code   **716.97 osteoarthritis, ankle**

INDICATIONS

- painful ankle, not responsive to medical and orthosis management; an intact joint space is a prerequisite (contraindicated in endstage arthritis)

ALTERNATIVE TREATMENTS

- ankle–foot orthosis (AFO), Arizona brace, NSAIDs, and corticosteroid or Hyalgan/Synvisc injections

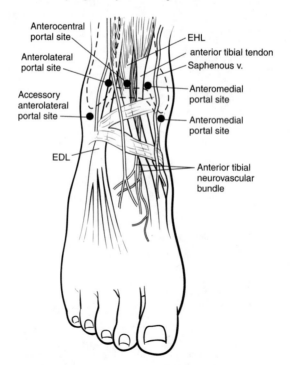

SURGICAL ANATOMY

- the topographic anatomy for the arthroscopy portals and their relationship to the anterior tibial tendon, neurovascular bundle, and the superficial peroneal nerve

Incision
- antcromedial portal just medial to the anterior tibial tendon
- anterolateral portal lateral to the superior peroneal nerve and extensor digitorum communis tendons

APPROACHES

Surgical Techniques
- the setup should have the knee flexed with the foot suspended free using a noninvasive distractor and heel strap; a high-flow inflow is used as well
- the 2.7-mm short 30° arthroscope and 2.9-mm shaver, as well as small arthroscopy instruments are part of the armamentarium; anterior capsule of the distal tibia and spurs are removed; the gutters and posterior joint are also visualized and debrided as needed (PRN)

POSTOPERATIVE MANAGEMENT

- posterior splint and non-weight-bearing for 1 week; portal sutures are removed at 7–10 days

REHABILITATION

- ROM and strengthening

COMPLICATIONS

- neuritis, 10%

SELECTED REFERENCE

Ferkel RD, Cheng JC. Ankle and subtalar arthroscopy. In: Kelikian AS, ed. Operative treatment of the foot and ankle. Stamford, CT: Appleton & Lange, 1999:321–350.

INDEX